What Leading Doctors and Health Care Professionals are saying about Darrell Stoddard and *Pain Free for Life*

I continue to be astonished at how dramatically and completely Darrell can get rid of severe pain. I have seen with my own eyes thousands of people becoming completely pain free when they thought they would have to live with pain the rest of their lives. ...This book contains many important ideas for enhanced health and well being. They are founded on the basis of published medical literature, and I believe are sound concepts.

— Dennis W. Remington, M.D., P.C.

Deafferentation, neurogenic pain—which is the most treatment resistant, is due to loss of neurologic signal from the periphery due to conduction loss—both neuropathic and tissue "volume conduction" changes. Stoddard's concept of reconnecting the system by use of conductive tape is a philosophical and practical "out of the box" end run for pain therapy.

—R. P. Iacono, M.D. FACS
Neuroscience/Neurosurgery

Dr. Iacono is the leading neurosurgeon that pioneered Sterotactic Pallidotomy brain surgery for Parkinson's disease.

Darrell Stoddard presents information that when accepted and implemented *will change the way modern medicine treats pain*. Everyone suffering from pain will benefit.

— Kent Pendleton, Health Educator

I am pleased to recommend Darrell Stoddard's book *Pain Free for Life* that provides a valid, low-risk, low-cost, alternative to modern medicine's drug and surgery approach to pain. Darrell's work is based on many years of hands-on experience with thousands of people. He has demonstrated that his simple, non-invasive treatments cannot only relieve pain quickly, but actually stop the cause of pain. Medical practitioners would do well to incorporate his methods as a first response for dealing with pain.

— Mark C. Belk, Ph.D.

Since I began using Biotape 5 years ago I would say that it gives great results 90% of the time. I have sent it home with many patients with the instruction to apply it where it hurts! It always works within a few minutes to an hour and usually within a few days the disability is gone.

— John E. Gambee, M.D.

This book presents a 180-degree paradigm shift from the drug based pharmaceutical approach of managing pain, to treating the cause of pain. It is "outside the box" thinking that should be considered by every medical doctor.

—David Voss, D.O.

I have watched Darrell work and produce dramatic pain relief for my wife. We had one of his machines in our home for a number of years and I was able to relieve my wife's pain and that of many others.

— A. Owen Smoot M.D., Orthopedic Surgeon

PAIN FREE
For Life

How to Heal Yourself
Naturally without Drugs
or Surgery

DARRELL STODDARD

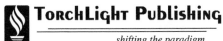

TorchLight Publishing

shifting the paradigm

AN IMPORTANT NOTE:

The ideas, positions, and statements in this book may in some cases conflict with orthodox, mainstream medical opinion, and the advice regarding health matters outlined in this book is not suitable for everyone. Do not attempt self-diagnosis, and do not embark upon self-treatment of any kind without qualified medical supervision. Nothing in this book should be construed as a promise of benefits or of results to be achieved, or a guarantee by the author or publisher of the safety or efficacy of its contents. The author, the publisher, its editors, and its employees disclaim any liability, loss, or risk incurred directly or indirectly as a result of the use or application of any of the contents of this book. If you are not willing to be bound by this disclaimer, please return your copy of the book to the publisher for a full refund.

First Printing 2003

Cover and Interior design by Mayapriya Long, Bookwrights Design

Printed in the United States of America

Published simultaneously in the United States of America and Canada by Torchlight Publishing.

Library of Congress Cataloging-in-Publication Data

Stoddard, Darrell J., 1934-
 Pain free for life : how to heal yourself naturally without drugs or
surgery / Darrell J Stoddard.
    p. cm.
Includes bibliographical references.
 ISBN 1-887089-46-2
 1. Pain—Popular works. 2. Pain—Alternative treatment. 3.
Medicine,
Chinese. I. Title.
RB127 .S775 2003
616'.0472—dc21

                    2003000629

Attention Colleges, Universities, Corporations, Associations and Professional Organizations: *Pain Free for Life* is available at special discounts for bulk purchases for training, sales promotions, premiums, fund-raising or educational use. Special books, booklets, or excerpts can be created to suit your specific needs.

For information contact the Publisher:

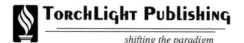 TorchLiqHt PublishiNq

shifting the paradigm

PO Box 52, Badger CA 93603
Phone: (559) 337-2200 • Fax: (559) 337-2354
Email: *torchlight@spiralcomm.net* • *www.torchlight.com*

—

Dedication

"Every man is a creature of the age in which he lives;
only a few are able to raise themselves
above the ideas of the time."

—Voltaire

This book is dedicated to medical saviors, the men and women below who made breakthroughs that will change the world forever, who challenged medical orthodoxy to raise themselves above the ideas of their time. All had their discoveries rejected. Most have been maligned. Revealing new truths, each stands alone. They have no peers.

Ignaz Philipp Semmelweis ⬦ Joseph Lister ⬦ William Harvey ⬦ James Lind ⬦ Edward Jenner ⬦ Samuel Smiles ⬦ Weston Price ⬦ Otto Warburg ⬦ Thomas McPherson Brown ⬦ Arthur Snow ⬦ Johanna Budwig ⬦ Oliver Sachs ⬦ Joseph Price ⬦ Paul Nogier ⬦ Deepak Chopra ⬦ John Gofman ⬦ George Meinig ⬦ F. Batmanghelidj ⬦ Alfred Nickel ⬦ Robert P. Iacono ⬦ Mary Enig ⬦ William B. Grant ⬦ Jerome Sullivan ⬦ Jukka Salonen ⬦ Joseph Mercola ⬦ David W. Gregg ⬦ Hunter "Patch" Adams ⬦ Dennis Remington ⬦ Gary and Victoria Beck, parents of autistic child Parker Beck, featured on *Dateline* October 7, 1998 ⬦ Sydney Ross Singer and Soma Grismaijer (authors of *Dressed to Kill*) ⬦ Augusto and Michaela Odone, (Lorenzo's real parents, not the actors, from the motion picture, *Lorenzo's Oil*)

"All great concepts that are currently accepted by those
who criticize were initially vigorously opposed
by their predecessors."

—Robert Barefoot

Contents

CHAPTER FIVE
More Preventable Causes of Pain (Fibromyalgia, Chronic Fatigue Syndrome, and Alzheimer's Disease)   101

CHAPTER SIX
Conclusion   119

Appendixes   127

Acknowledgments

*"The problems of the world cannot possibly
be solved by skeptics or cynics whose
horizons are limited by obvious realities.
We need men who can dream of things
that never were and ask, 'Why not?'"*

—Spencer W. Kimball

My *impossible dream* is **to change the way Western
medicine defines and treats pain.** A corollary to my impossible dream is the preposterous claim that **Western medicine
has never defined what pain is** (a definition the Chinese
have known for two thousand years). I don't expect anyone
to believe the dream possible. You, my reader, will have to
decide whether or not *Western medicine has ever defined
what pain is* by finding answers to your own pain.

I'm spurred on to do the impossible by four of my
running companions: Peter Strudwick, who has run more
than sixty 26-mile marathons without feet; Harry Cordellos,
who is totally blind and holds world records and has won
gold medals in distance running, swimming, cycling, and
cross-country skiing; George Murray, world champion
wheelchair athlete, who in three months wheeled a wheelchair from the ocean in San Diego to the ocean on the coast
of Maine; and Larry Lewis, who at 103 ran six miles every
morning before going to work.

My son taught me that it is possible for a human to ride a bicycle more than 1200 miles in twenty-four hours, or to ride a bicycle 152 miles per hour *if someone or something goes before them* to overcome wind resistance (drafting). Mike Sechrist and John Howard actually set these records on bicycles. Have you ever driven a *car* 152 miles an hour or 1200 miles in twenty-four hours?

Those behind whom I have *drafted,* who have gone before me to make this book possible and to make me think I can do the impossible are: My still living ninety-six-year-old mother, who reads my manuscripts and thinks they are wonderful; my father, who, with his eighth-grade education taught me two of the most important medical truths I know; my wife, because she let me come back to bed after I got up to write in the middle of the night; my children and grand-children, who are my motivation for writing; my brother Lynn, for his encouragement; Pattie, for editing help; Kenneth Cooper, M.D., for teaching me about heart disease and aerobics; Arthur Snow, M.D., for teaching me the cause of all degenerative disease; Daniel Kirsch, for inventing the wonderful instrument I use and for teaching me electromedicine; Dr. Zhang Le Pei, for teaching me Chinese auricular medi-cine; Terry Oleson for his book and epoch work in Auriculotherapy; Gaston Naessons and Walter Clifford, for teaching me about the miracle of live blood; George Meinig, DDS, for teaching me about root canals; Dennis Remington, M.D., who has an open mind and who let me practice my strange Chinese craft for thirteen years although we were called quacks; Kent Pendleton, medical educator, who knows more about how the body works than anyone; Joanna Budwig, my mentor and advisor; Robert Iacono, M.D. neurosurgeon, who read my papers and agreed with me about the cause of pain; John Gofman, M.D., who revealed to me the almost unknown cause of most cancer and who has defended my work; my patients, who let me practice on them and somehow miraculously got better; Bob Tisman and Tonda Mullis, my advocates; Alister Taylor, my publisher, who sees the big picture; the Tic Tack Toe Chicken at the Texas State Fair that keeps me humble; last, and most important, are the nameless Chinese who two thousand years ago discovered that "pain and disease are caused by the blockage of chi and the stagnation of blood."

"In great attempts, it is glorious even to fail"

—Longinus

Foreword

I first met Darrell Stoddard about fourteen years ago. He walked into the office, all sweaty, in jogging attire, saying that he had been out for a run when he went by our office and recognized my name. He had heard another doctor severely criticizing me, and wondered what kind of a doctor would produce so much anger and animosity in another doctor. Over the years I had integrated a variety of alternative and complementary techniques into my family practice, and at the time, I was seriously considering buying an electrical stimulation instrument for pain I had seen demonstrated. I told Darrell this, and he then described a therapeutic instrument he was using to stimulate acupuncture points on the ears for pain control. I was intrigued by this new concept Darrell described, especially since it involved acupuncture technology. We scheduled a time for him to demonstrate his instrument a few days later on patients with pain. Most of these people underwent such dramatic pain relief that we then arranged for Darrell to come into the office full-time to treat our patients.

Ever since that day, Darrell has been with us, and that has been our good fortune (although he has recently become semi-retired and is now only working one day a week).

I continue to be astonished at how dramatically and completely Darrell can free people from severe pain. I have physically seen thousands of people becoming completely pain free—people who thought they would live with pain for the rest of their lives. I remember one man in particular. He had been totally disabled by a car accident he was in over forty years previously. Fractures in his neck, back, and right wrist had left severe residual pain. He had come to see me for help with abdominal pain; he was taking so many painkillers, and they were irritating his stomach. He was skeptical when I described the pain therapy, and I had to talk hard to get him to try it. Even then he was only willing to have his neck treated. When one treatment completely eradicated the neck pain, he could hardly wait to come back and get the other areas treated. His pain disappeared completely after each area was treated.

It has been frustrating over my years of medical practice not to have been able to alleviate most kinds of pain. Usually, we are able to simply control the symptoms of pain with drugs and surgery. Drugs control symptoms at best, but most often do that poorly. They also have a lot of side effects. All effective painkillers are addictive, and I hate to see people struggling with addiction. Surgery is often ineffective too, and regularly creates new pains often worse than the original reason for which the surgery was done! It is exciting to be able to control pain with a technique that not only works a lot better than the options but is frequently curative as well. Healing regularly occurs when energetic pathways are opened and the cause of the pain is addressed. All of this has been possible without expensive, dangerous drugs or painful surgery!

Not only has Darrell's treatment worked well for pain, it has also been effective for restoring function in a lot of other medical conditions. Conditions such as tremors, depression, stress incontinence, and others are helped when the acupuncture points are electrically stimulated.

Darrell has an insatiable curiosity. He reads widely and is a creative thinker. I have had the opportunity to read much of what he has written about a variety of medical issues. He has a strong desire to help people, and has gathered together a compilation of helpful measures that should help people prevent and treat health problems. I was delighted when Darrell told me he was putting a lot of these ideas into a book.

The book before you contains a lot of Darrell's important ideas for enhanced health and well-being. They are based on published medical literature and I believe they are sound concepts. Only further research will prove whether all of the theories presented in this book are correct. Still, I would like to encourage any medical professional who reads this book to read with an open mind and not to reject the concepts for lack of such proof. Keep in mind that at least eighty to ninety percent of everything traditional medical doctors do has not been proven by prospective, randomized, double blind studies or other types of acceptable research.

Darrell has a real gift for healing. Unfortunately, not everyone can receive direct, hands-on treatment from him. The innovations he has made can be helpful, however. I certainly have been impressed with the results of the bioelectric materials he has developed. We use these materials in our office, and I have seen them dramatically eliminate pain and promote healing.

I would like to encourage readers of this book to make some of the changes in lifestyle Darrell has recommended. Eat a healthy diet, drink plenty of clean, safe water, and apply other healthy lifestyle changes. These can promote huge improvements on the road to optimal health.

Dennis W. Remington, M.D., P.C.

PAIN FREE
For Life

Introduction

"There is nothing more difficult to take in hand, more perilous to conduct, or more uncertain in its success, than to take the lead in the introduction of a new order of things."

—Nicolo Machiavelli

Teaching you how to be pain free for life is the purpose of this book. To do this, the book must reveal precisely what pain is. It must teach you *how* to prevent and heal pain naturally, without drugs or surgery. The book must also be true to the Hippocratic Oath, which states, "… and I will abstain from all intentional wrongdoing and harm… "

Because there are millions of people in pain, and because pain medications are harmful, the above goals are obviously not known, observed, or practiced. To even suggest that modern medicine does not know what pain is or how to treat it without doing harm is preposterous. How could that be? I don't expect you to believe even the possibility that modern medicine could be so profoundly wrong without considering the following recent catastrophic medical mistakes:

Prescribing thalidomide to prevent morning sickness. This caused thousands of babies to be born deformed.

Randolph Warren, 37, CEO of the Thalidomide Victims Association of Canada, reported that his mother took two tablets of the drug prescribed to prevent morning sickness and that he was born with deformed arms and legs. "I had twenty-four operations before the age of sixteen," he said. "That's what just two doses of Thalidomide can do." There are more than 5,000 surviving Thalidomide babies in the world today.

Not challenging the health effect of cigarettes, or the ad, "More Doctors Smoke Camels Than Any Other Brand." "More Doctors Smoke Camels Than Any Other Brand" was the byline for a multitude of ads that appeared for more than a decade in *all* national publications (with *Reader's Digest* as the one exception.) The ads were unchallenged by the American Medical Association for years because, at that time, many doctors *did* smoke.

Failing to recognize that folic acid prevents neural tube birth defects. It took the FDA more than thirty years to even acknowledge that folic acid prevents neural tube birth defects. Thousands of deformed babies were born because the FDA prohibited claims that pregnant women should take folic acid. Now such information is accepted, recommended, and widely publicized.

The above medical mistakes are well known, but almost as catastrophic and unknown is:

Radiating millions of children in the '30s and '40s with X-rays for an "enlarged thymus" to prevent congestion. We now know that an enlarged thymus is part of a normal child's development and a manifestation of a healthy immune system. *The X-radiation of so many* *children with an enlarged thymus is unquestionably the cause of much of the cancer we are seeing today.* Such X-ray treatments and many other such uses of X-rays (Roentgen therapy) have been totally stopped (along with X-ray machines in department stores to fit shoes) because of the cancer they caused. Few in the medical field will even talk about the harmful use of X-rays in the past because X-rays are still being used in medicine today. (See: *Better Than a Cure for Breast Cancer* by the author of this book at *http://www.healpain.net*.)

A catastrophic medical mistake that has been totally and quietly stopped is:

Putting Merthiolate or Mercurochrome on every cut, scrape, burn, or wound in America, and using Merthiolate or Mercurochrome to swab sore throats. Did it stop sore throats or infection? Yes, incredibly well. Merthiolate or Mercurochrome were marvelous disinfectants; they killed *all* the bacteria and *all* the germs. The reason these products are no longer used or even on the market today is that the "Mer" in Merthiolate and Mercurochrome is MERCURY, one of the most toxic substances on earth.

More recent catastrophic medical mistakes include:

Prescribing Fen-phen to lose weight. This caused heart valve damage in thousands of patients.

Prescribing Prempro (Premarin and Proverra) **for hormone replacement.** Prempro increased risk of breast cancer by 26 percent, and raised the number of strokes by 41 percent and the number of heart attacks by 29 percent. A 16,600-patient study, which lasted over five years and was supposed to continue until 2005, was abruptly halted in late May (2002) after researchers found that the newly identified risks of taking the drug outweighed its benefits.

Performing 650,000 arthroscopic surgeries each year for osteoarthritis of the knee—surgeries that are no better than a placebo according to the July 11, 2001 *New England Journal of Medicine.* Traditional Western medicine prides itself in doing only that which has been scientifically validated by randomized blind or double blind placebo-controlled crossover studies. No surgical procedures currently being performed (with the exception of the one above) have ever been subjected to placebo-controlled studies. Is it possible that other surgical procedures will prove to be "no better than a placebo" if they are subjected to the scrutiny of placebo-controlled studies? (See Chapter Two.)

An almost unknown but still catastrophic medical mistake is:

Failing to recognize the negative health effects of root canal infections, even when the infection does not show up on an X-ray. In the '30s and '40s when people were sick, sick, sick, we would pull all of their teeth and they would get better. Now we save the teeth no matter what and have millions of chronically ill patients. No one is able to determine the cause of their illness. If you or a loved one is seriously ill and no one can help, read *A Healing Miracle from Relentless Pain Caused by a Root Canal* at: *http:// www.healpain.net.* The story is important, because root canal infections—something the immune system cannot heal—may be the cause of inscrutable pain or chronic illness, pain or illness modern medicine will not be able to help until the cause is recognized.

A current medical practice that is a catastrophic medical mistake is:

The unlimited use of fluoroscopic X-ray examinations where the x-ray beam remains on. All medical doctors (and everyone else) is concerned about whether or not mammograms cause cancer. Many studies and most doctors would concede that old mammography instruments (which exposed patients to ten times the radiation as the new low-dose instruments) did indeed cause some cancer. That is why so much has been done to reduce the dose. New digital instruments (much better even than low-dose mammography) have reduced the dose by almost one hundred times. Still, no one even blinks an eye at the unlimited use of fluoroscopic X-ray examinations that may expose patients to two hundred times as much radiation as low-dose mammography and a thousand times more radiation than the new digital mammography instruments. This is not "gagging on a gnat and swallowing a camel." It is "gagging on a gnat and swallowing a herd of elephants." (See: *A Major Cause of Cancer and Heart Disease, Your Doctor, Dentist, or Chiropractor Does Not Want You To Know* at *http://www.healpain.net.*)

I compare fluoroscopy to swallowing a *herd* of elephants (instead of a single elephant) because fluoroscopy is not rare. It is one of the most common X-ray procedures performed, and is used many times daily in every hospital in America. Still, less than one percent of the population (aside from medical professionals) even knows what fluoroscopy is.

Other catastrophic medical mistakes include:

Treating depression with anti-depressant drugs. This is wrong because they have harmful side effects, they do not cure the problem, and because there is a better way. (See: *Depression Cure* at *http://www.healpain.net.*)

Abandoning the theory that aluminum is one of the causes of Alzheimer's disease. There is compelling *new* evidence that aluminum is not only a major cause of Alzheimer's but fibromyalgia and chronic fatigue syndrome as well. (See Chapter Five.)

This brings us to the subject of this book: pain and how pain is treated. This also brings us to what may be another catastrophic medical mistake:

Treating pain with pain medication. Every pain medication used is a violation of the Hippocratic Oath, because every pain medication has harmful side effects and may even cause death. This includes all over-the-counter pain medications (known as NSAIDs—non-steroidal anti-inflammatory drugs), acetaminophen (Tylenol™), and prescription steroids and narcotics.

Treating pain with pain medication is also profoundly wrong because you are treating the symptom and not the cause. Pain is a protective device; it protects us from further injury. When we suppress the pain signal with *any* kind of pain medication, we lose the protection pain gives. We in the West are stuck in a lose-lose situation when treating our pain because Western medicine has never defined exactly what pain is. When we don't know what pain is, we can only "manage" it, or treat the pain symptom.

Is it incomprehensible that Western medicine does not know what pain is? The International Association for the Study of Pain defines pain as "an unpleasant sensory and emotional experience associated with actual or potential tissue damage." This tells us little about the physiology of pain, nothing about how the body heals pain, and absolutely nothing about how to treat pain.

One of the purposes of this book is to challenge the way Western medicine defines and treats pain by revealing what causes pain and how to scientifically validate, with a double-blind placebo-controlled study, exactly what pain is—something the Chinese have known for two thousand years. The failure of Western medicine to properly investigate the Chinese definition of pain has kept us from learning what pain is. Instead, we call pain a symptom, then treat the symptom and not the cause with harmful drugs or surgery. Why haven't we seriously considered the Chinese theory of pain?

Evidences that Western medicine has never investigated the Chinese definition of pain are statements such as the following (such statements can be found on hundreds of medical websites): "No one knows why acupuncture works. We think it may work by releasing endorphins in the brain."

While this may be true, the *real* reason acupuncture works can be learned simply by asking the Chinese medical doctors. Acupuncture works because it reconnects the broken Chi. A well known TV series claimed, "No one has ever seen or measured Chi." This is wrong. I have measured Chi in more than eighteen thousand patients. Chi is not a mystery. *Chi is the endogenous electrical signals in living tissue that can be measured and quantified.* "Broken Chi" is the cause of all acute and chronic pain.

Compelling evidence that Chinese medical theory may be correct appeared in an announcement by the U.S. Food and Drug Administration on April 19, 1999, approving an electricity test to detect breast cancer. The announcement described how the test worked: "A one-volt shot of electricity is sent into the hand, where it travels through the body into the breast. A handheld probe is moved over the breast, where it measures the electrical conductivity of breast cells. Cancer cells conduct *much* less electricity than healthy cells, so when the probe flashes its findings onto a computer screen, possible tumors show up as bright white spots."

In Chinese medicine there is only one diagnosis: the blockage of Chi. The blockage of Chi refers to *unhealthy cells conducting much less electricity than healthy cells.* Where there is breast cancer, *cells conduct much less electricity than healthy cells.* Where there is pain, *cells conduct much less electricity than healthy cells.* (We wonder how many other kinds of cancer and disease will prove to *conduct much less electricity than healthy cells.*) These are demonstrable medical facts confirming Chinese medical theory. It will take a paradigm shift in our thinking, but Western medicine must learn these facts and apply them before it will be able to deal effectively with pain or cancer.

The goal of this book is to reveal a better way to treat pain without drugs or surgery. Knowing what causes pain allows us not to manage but heal pain and thus become pain-free for life.

❧

"Scientific proof that does not conform to the establishment's preconceived concepts is always rejected initially."

—Robert Barefoot

—

CHAPTER ONE

The Real Cause of Pain

Why it still hurts when the doctor can find nothing wrong

"Pain can be a more terrible lord of mankind than even death himself."

—Albert Schweitzer

ABSTRACT

Failure to Define What Pain Is. Pharmaceutical Treatments for Pain. Surgery for Pain. Exercise as a Treatment for Pain. What Pain Is (as opposed to what is thought to cause pain). Bioelectric and Auricular Therapy (treating pain without drugs, surgery, or exercise). Case Studies (from more than 18,000 treatments). Is it Anecdotal or Placebo? When Bioelectric and Auricular Therapy Do Not Work. Has Electrical Stimulation Been Proven? Summary on Treating Pain.

13

Failure to Define What Pain Is

How can people have severe pain when they have not been injured and the most sophisticated imaging devices find nothing wrong? Why are other people pain-free, even when they have conditions said to cause pain? Maybe we don't know what pain is or what causes it. I submit that pain is more than a symptom.

For me to suggest that pain be treated as a disease instead of a symptom is like Galileo claiming that the earth revolves around the sun. Everyone knew he was wrong. They simply had to look up in the sky and see the sun going around the earth for themselves. Everyone knows that injury causes pain. Thus pain is nothing but a signal that something is wrong, a sign of injury. This interpretation (a mindset cast in stone) has prevented Western medicine from defining or learning what pain is. Calling pain a symptom and believing that it is beneficial because it helps us with diagnosis, tells us only what pain does, not what it is. As the earth revolves around the sun, there is a better understanding of and way to deal with pain.

Numerous studies have been done on how pain signals are transmitted to the brain. It has been found that endogenous neuroactive substances (endorphins and encephalins) in the brain and spinal column control our perception of pain. Science has discovered that chemicals named prostaglandin and bradykinin are released in the body when we are injured, but none of the studies adequately defines pain. Neither the mechanism of transmission, how the brain deals with pain, nor the chemical response to pain, actually tells us what pain *is*.

We claim that pain is caused by injury, inflammation, infection, pinched nerves, nerve damage, herniated discs, bone spurs, arthritis, rheumatism, scar tissue, adhesions, fractures, torn cartilage, torn ligaments, bone on bone due to worn out cartilage, etc. Logically, this is the same as saying that drinking water causes pain, since everyone who has pain drinks water. The fact is, not everyone who drinks water does have pain. Similarly, not everyone with any of the above purported causes of pain suffers pain.

Three personal examples:

Example 1: My oldest son had a high school wrestling injury and had surgery in which all of the cartilage in his knee was removed. His knee is now bone on bone, yet he still runs twenty-six-mile marathons, rides a two hundred-mile bike race every year, and recently set a record for cycling 334 miles across Utah—more than twenty-four hours of continuous hard riding. He experienced no knee pain! Does bone on bone cause pain? No!

Example 2: My son-in-law's arm was dragged into a piece of farm machinery when he was a boy. The arm was terribly crushed. Skilled surgeons saved his arm, but today it is almost solid scar tissue. Still he has no pain. Does scar tissue cause pain? No!

Example 3: A few years ago I spoke at the funeral of a woman who had lost more than six inches of her height due to vertebral compression fractures. Almost all of her thoracic vertebrae were fractured, but she repeatedly said she never had back pain. Do compression fractures cause pain? No!

What about pinched nerves? Are they a cause of pain? The July 14, 1994 *New England Journal of Medicine* reported a study showing MRI total spine scans performed on ninety-eight adults without back pain. Sixty-four percent of these adults, it turned out, had some type of disc abnormality (herniation), and thirty-eight percent had abnormalities in two or more discs. Do herniated discs pressing on nerves cause pain? No! Neither do any of the other conditions Western medicine gives as causes of pain. If those conditions in themselves caused pain, everyone *with* those conditions would experience pain, and that is simply not true.

Nerves can function perfectly without pain even when they are pinched. The reverse is also true. Patients can have severe pain even without nerve compression. Imaging devices (X-rays, CT scans, and MRIs) may show where a nerve is pinched without telling anything about the signal traveling through the nerve.

Even torn rotator cuffs do not cause pain. University of Miami researchers performed MRIs on the dominant shoulder of ninety-six people with no history of shoulder pain. Thirty-four percent had at least partial tears of the rotator cuff. More than half of the subjects over sixty had rotator cuff tears. None of them had pain.

Severe crippling rheumatoid arthritis does not cause pain. The reason I can make such an extreme statement is because people with rheumatoid arthritis do not hurt all the time (even when their pain is not masked by medication). If the arthritis was causing the pain, they would experience pain twenty-four hours a day every day. Arthritis pain goes up and down; there are times when it flares up, and periods in which the sufferer is relatively pain free. If the arthritis caused the pain, the pain would never stop, because the twisted, swollen joints do not come and go. They are present whether or not the pain is flaring up or not present. For these reasons, we know that something that goes with the arthritis is causing the pain, not the arthritis itself.

Why has American medicine never discovered what pain is? Why has it failed to define pain? It has failed because we pride ourselves on treating "causes," not symptoms, and pain is never thought of as anything other than a symptom. Thus the cause of pain is not studied.

Anesthesiologist John J. Bonica, founder of the International Association for the Study of Pain, surveyed seventeen standard textbooks used in medical schools and found that only fifty-four pages out of a total twenty thousand even mentioned the word "pain." Less than one percent of the medical school curriculum addresses pain, even though pain is the single-most common reason people take medication or see a doctor. "Chronic pain disables more people than cancer or heart disease," Bonica writes, "and it costs the American people more money than both."

Even the celebrated "Gate Theory of Pain" by Wall and Melzack is based on the assumption that pain is a symptom. Wall and Melzack discovered how pain signals are transmitted to the brain, not what pain is. Understanding the mechanism of pain transmission has value because we can learn how to block our perception of pain. Blocking the pain signal, however, does not "heal" what causes the pain.

The idea that pain is beneficial because it tells us something is wrong or helps us diagnose a problem has kept us from learning what pain is. Who needs the excruciating pain known as "tic-douloureux" (trigeminal neuralgia)? Do we need arthritis pain to diagnose crippling rheumatoid arthritis? Does fibromyalgia pain reveal an underlying pathology? No. As far as we know in these and a host of other infirmities, the pain is the disease. Pain may be beneficial, but more often than not, it serves no useful function.

A severe headache may lead to the discovery of a brain tumor, but what do we do for the millions of headache sufferers who don't have tumors? An equally difficult question: Why do some patients still have paralyzing back pain after surgery has apparently eliminated the cause? The pain reveals nothing. If all those with a condition we think should cause pain do not suffer pain, or if people have severe pain with no apparent cause, maybe that means we don't know what pain is or what causes it.

Pharmaceutical Treatments for Pain

We can eliminate pain in two ways: we can suppress our perception of pain with medication, or we can heal what is causing the pain. If we suppress the sensory nerves with medication, it will either cause gastrointestinal bleeding or suppressed motor, bowel, kidney, liver, respiratory, or mental function.

Is there a healthcare practitioner who has not seen cancer patients on morphine who have lost the use of their bowels or legs? Is it not the nerve suppression with drugs for pain rather than the cancer itself that causes constipation or loss of function? The body can heal pain without suppressive medication, but how?

Surgery for Pain

What about surgery aimed specifically at pain—cutting the nerve—in contrast to surgery aimed at correcting the condition thought to cause the pain? An article on pain in the June 11, 1984 issue of *Time* tells of a neurosurgeon who tries to talk people out of surgery for pain. He explains, "Although operations to destroy nerves can provide immediate relief, the benefits rarely last more than six months to a year and may be followed by an intense burning pain that is worse than the original complaint!"

Exercise as a Treatment for Pain

What else can be done for pain? "You can take drugs, have surgery, or exercise," is an answer I heard given at a spine center dedicated to treating chronic back pain. The practitioners said there were no other choices, but they were wrong.

If not drugs or surgery, then what about exercise? On November 2, 1994, CBS broadcast a one-hour special on pain treatments in which they first exposed a number of fraudulent pain practices. They then showed what was supposed to be a state-of-the-art pain treatment center affiliated with a well-known medical school that used exercise to treat pain. During the program, the doctor being interviewed explained that if you have pain from a broken ankle, exercise is harmful. For some types of chronic back pain, however, "exercising through the pain" is the best and perhaps only way to heal it. Patients were required to complete nineteen painful exercise sessions, which cost them more than $20,000. The patient featured on CBS was only able to complete thirteen or fourteen of these sessions before the pain was too much to endure. The insurance company paying for his treatments dropped him.

Exercise may be the best medicine for heart disease and a multitude of ailments, but it is a Catch-22 when we hurt too much to perform it. Exercise and other approaches to pain that require numerous treatments may simply be doing something we *think* is helpful, while the body heals itself in some unknown way. Neither does exercise directly address what we think causes pain or what pain is.

What Pain Is
(as opposed to what is thought to cause pain)

The need to deal with what pain *actually* is instead of what we think causes it is illustrated when we hit our thumb with a hammer. No one can argue that the hammer blow caused the pain. But that is a past event, one that cannot be changed. Now we must deal with what the pain is, not what we think caused it.

For us to understand what pain is instead of what we think causes pain, we must understand the body's electrophysiology. The body has millions of biologically closed electrical circuits.[1] These wonderfully tuned and balanced circuits connect virtually all of the body's cells.

It is erroneous to think that electricity travels only through nerves. Blood and blood vessels are also conductors. Electricity travels through arteries, veins, capillaries, muscles, tendons, ligaments, lymphatic vessels, and bones. Every living cell has an electrical potential, and many, if not all, bodily functions are controlled electrically.

Another factor we need to understand about the electrical circulatory system is how delicately it is balanced. Just touching someone and holding pressure can reduce the electrical resistance by as much as two hundred percent, thereby increasing the flow of the body's endogenous electrical signals (a phenomenon that can be measured and quantified). This is why touch heals, massage is therapeutic, and babies have to be held, touched, caressed, and cuddled to develop normally. This is why acupuncture and acupressure work. Just putting an acupuncture needle in the body can dramatically decrease the resistance and increase the flow of electricity. This is why nerve conduction tests in which needles are inserted along dermatomes (nerve pathways) to measure nerve signals invalidates what we measure simply by inserting the needles.

When we look only for what we think causes pain instead of dealing with what pain is, there are as many different prescribed treatments as there are causes. If we deal with what pain is, then the same treatment would be helpful no matter what we think causes the pain.

Doctors have been trying for more than two hundred years to find out what causes pain without ever learning what pain is. If we don't know what pain is, all we can do is suppress our symptoms and hope the body heals itself.

We tend to give medications that only mask pain, suppress vital functions, or cause gastrointestinal bleeding. If we can't find anything wrong, we imply that the pain is in the patient's head or tell them they have to learn to live with the pain. Others are sent to surgery or endless therapy with astronomical costs. By the end, the patient may be in worse pain than before he started.

Everyone knows that injury causes pain, but what is the cause of pain when there has been no injury? Pain may continue long after an injury takes place. Why does it still hurt? What exactly is pain? How does the body heal pain?

We are aware of the sensation of touch because when we are touched, our cells are pushed closer together. This decreases the electrical resistance between cells. Decreasing the electrical resistance increases the electrical signal going to the brain. The increased flow of electricity is what tells us that we have been touched.

When something hits us, it sends a quick burst of electricity to the brain. If pain continues after the blow, it is because tissue has been damaged and electrical connections between cells have been broken. The brain senses the injury because of a signal from the damaged tissue to the brain. The pain signal, however, is not the pain! In reality, pain is broken or suppressed electrical signals between cells in the injured tissue.

What about pain that is not caused by injury? Degenerative diseases, dehydration, inflammation, infection, ulcers, tumors, lack of minerals, spontaneous fractures, allergies, etc., may also cause the electrical circuits to fail, even when there has been no injury. Whether it is that injury has broken the electrical circuits or those signals have failed for some other reason, the signal to the brain is the same. Both are interpreted as pain.

The failure of electrical connections between cells is not only the cause of pain but also the cause of all degenerative diseases according to Traditional Chinese medicine. The theory is not so incredulous when we know that the brain works electrically and that we are "brain dead" when there is no more electricity going across our brain. All cells will die or become degenerate if electrical signals are broken or suppressed.

If pain is the breaking, suppression, or failure of the body's electrical circuits, how does the body heal pain? Pain is healed when the body *reconnects* the broken circuits. When we hit our thumb with a hammer, it hurts because electrical connections between the cells have been broken. It stops hurting when the body reconnects the broken circuits. This is the way the body heals pain, and the only way it heals pain—by finding and reconnecting the broken circuits.

Does this definition apply to any and all kinds of pain? Yes. Is there a method that will relieve pain, chronic as well as acute, often with only one treatment? Yes. Did I discover it? No. Is it a new discovery? No. It is, in fact, more than

2000 years old. Traditional Chinese medicine defines pain as a "stagnation of blood" or a "blockage of Chi." This could be interpreted as an interruption or blockage of the body's electrical circuits. If the Chinese are correct and my interpretation is accurate, then pain is something that can be measured and quantified. Western medicine says that pain can neither be measured nor quantified, but Western medicine is wrong.

Bioelectric and Auricular Therapy
(treating pain without drugs, surgery, or exercise)

How do you treat broken or suppressed electrical circuits to restore and maintain electrical conductivity? Not by putting on TENS (transcutaneous electronic nerve stimulation) pads and turning up the power to block or override the pain signal. Rather, first you need to use an instrument that measures the resistance before and after the stimulation cycle to gather the following information: to find where the circuits are suppressed, to know how long to stimulate, and to determine when the desired results have been achieved. To be effective, the instrument must deliver a biologically compatible current in the microampere (millionths of an amp) range at or near the levels of the body's own electrical functions. I have named this more discriminating approach to electrical stimulation "bioelectric therapy" in contrast to the TENS. (Most TENS units differ from my bioelectric therapy instrument, in that they are in the milliampere range, which is one thousand times more powerful.

Traditional acupuncture has presented evidence that it is able to turn on broken circuits, but it cannot accurately measure the results. Acupuncture, like many other pain therapies, also requires multiple treatments. What is needed is not simply something to turn on the failed circuits but something to keep them turned on so that the pain will not return. (Patented Biotape™ from the Pain Research Institute will do this. See Chapter Three.)

Traditional Chinese medicine provides both an answer and a method. Auricular therapy (ear acupuncture performed without needles) stimulates acupuncture points by taping tiny seeds on combinations of the 136 identified points in each ear. You may know about acupuncture anesthesia, where major operations are performed with out anesthesia or pain. For chronic conditions, auricular therapy is better than acupuncture, because with one treatment, pressure from the seeds continues twenty-four hours a day for up to one month. This is better than receiving acupuncture with needles every day. The constant, twenty-four-hour pressure from the seeds stimulates the corresponding centers in the brain to keep the broken circuits turned on. "Healing" is thus achieved. With this method, the patient does not have to return again and again to get results, and the pain often does not return either.

The body heals pain through the brain rather than by pharmacological methods that only suppress the pain signal (along with other vital functions). Does defining and stopping pain this way sound too good to be true? Below are case studies using this treatment on patients with severe, chronic, and intractable pain.

Case Studies
(from more than eighteen thousand treatments)

Patient David M.: Severe pain in neck and shoulders, fingers numb. MRI showed degenerative cervical disc disease with nerve root impairment. Major surgery was scheduled for the following Wednesday. Patient received almost total relief of pain with first treatment before leaving treatment room. Surgery was canceled. One month later and one treatment later, all of the feeling returned to his hand. Three months after first treatment, pain gone completely and full function and feeling in hand. No treatment needed. Insurance company distressed because David is not following doctors' orders. (Those who watch the bottom line in the company need to realize that the insurance company saved the cost of surgery and did not even have to pay for the treatment!)

Patient Orvil E.: "Suicidal" cluster (Migrainous Neuralgia) headaches for more than forty years. Saw untold numbers of doctors, neurologists, headache specialists, etc., including doctors at the Mayo Clinic. None of them could provide anything but temporary relief. One treatment and patient has now gone for more than two years without medication or headaches.

Patient Mike W.: Serious back injury. Surgery, then after surgery, intractable, disabling, "inoperable" pain. On more than one occasion patient went to gun closet to end pain. With his finger on the trigger, he realized he couldn't go through with it because of his family. Pain disappeared with first treatment. Had two more treatments just to make sure pain would not return. No more back pain until back was reinjured. With one treatment patient is again functional and almost pain-free.

Patient Julia J.: Scheduled for nerve root decompression cervical surgery. One treatment and the pain went away. Surgery canceled. Patient now able to "quilt all day without pain, which would have been impossible before." Still better without surgery five years later.

Patient Travis B.: Told he would be paralyzed if he didn't have lumbar surgery. One treatment and patient is fully functional with almost no pain for more than a year.

Post-surgical pain that resists every known treatment can also be helped. Patient Una H. was in constant pain and unable to function after spinal surgery. She attended a state-of-the-art spine center for therapy three times a week for more than six months. This didn't help, so she went to another spine center for three more months. She became worse. One treatment relieved eighty percent of the pain and seventy-five percent of her depression. Her lower leg had been numb since before the surgery, but after only one treatment, the feeling began to return.

Patient Katherine K.: Sobbing with pain. Couldn't sit or stand. Went to emergency room three days prior to treatment where she was given "six shots of morphine in a half-hour period that didn't even touch the pain." Thirty-minute treatment and patient was pain-free. Went back to work the next day and is still pain-free nearly a year later.

Patient Edwin H.: Fell twelve stories in a construction accident and survived! Spine fractured in several places.

Foot and leg bones shattered. Three years later his nerves were so compromised a neurosurgeon said another surgery might leave him paralyzed. With onset of arthritis, patient was told pain would get worse. He received "at least thirty percent relief" with the first treatment. The second treatment was so successful that patient did not return for over a year. Then patient came in for pain in his shattered foot. No more treatments were needed for pain in the back.

Patient Alberta M.: Skin around opening of vagina cracked and bleeding. The area was so sensitive she could hardly stand to have her undergarments touch her. Numerous MDs and OB-Gyns prescribed hormone creams and other treatments, but nothing improved the situation. One treatment of three auricular seeds taped on her ear brought one hundred percent relief. The problem has not recurred even four months later with no further treatment.

Patient Myrna V.: Breast cancer, mastectomy, then metastasis of the cancer to the cervical region of the spine causing severe neck, shoulder, and arm pain. Each treatment relieved pain for one month or more. After four treatments for pain together with cancer treatments, a spinal bone scan showed no metastases and no cancer. No claim is made for what appears to be a remission of cancer, but we still wonder if relieving the pain affected the cancer. (Bjorn Nordenstrom, the famous Swedish radiologist who pioneered needle aspiration biopsies, was able to eliminate malignant lung tumors by stimulating the tumors with a direct electric current.)

Patient Wayne M.: "Not one day without serious back pain in more than forty years." One treatment eliminated ninety-five percent of the pain. A year later with no more treatments, pain has still not returned.

Patient Elaine M.: Born with a cord that was too short in one side of her neck, which prevented her from turning her head in both directions. After one treatment, she has been able to turn her head all the way in both directions for the first time in more than sixty-five years.

Do the treatments last? Patient Joy C. was sent home after spending two weeks in a hospital in Virginia, with a letter from a neurosurgeon that said decompression back surgery was imperative. Without surgery, he said, she would be paralyzed or at least spend the rest of her life in a wheelchair. She couldn't get off the floor when she called me for help. After only two treatments she has been pain-free for fourteen years.

Is it Anecdotal or Placebo?

Is my definition of pain and what causes it anecdotal? Yes. I arrived at the above thesis by observing more than eighteen thousand treatments for pain using the above method and technology. I am prepared to travel anywhere to teach or demonstrate this treatment's effectiveness. I will also submit to any double-blind study. Relief often comes so quickly that it can be demonstrated before an audience. To provide evidence for what I am saying, I would like to treat a number of patients with intractable pain who have already tried everything else, including surgery, or for whom surgery is the only hope. Unless the nerves are completely severed, one or two treatments can often bring a healing.

There is also hope of healing when the nerves have been severed. A whiplash patient, who had received a $60,000 insurance settlement based on a neurologist's sworn testimony that cervical nerves had been severed, came to see me. Such a large judgment was awarded because it was understood that the patient would be in pain for the rest of her life. Each treatment leaves the patient pain-free for six months to over a year.

Were the above cases successful because of the placebo effect? Everyone familiar with medical research and double-blind studies knows that between thirty and thirty-five percent of the patients will improve no matter what a doctor does, provided the patient believes in the treatment. To determine whether our successes were due to the placebo effect, we asked 104 successive patients to complete an evaluation form. By this we would know that if we had helped no more than thirty to thirty-five percent of them, our treatments were worthless.

The results follow:

If I am correct that pain is an interruption of the body's electrical circuits, then what causes the pain may also cause arthritis and other degenerative diseases instead of arthritis and other diseases being responsible for causing pain. In his book, *The Body Electric,* orthopedic

Results of 104 Successive Patients

100%	Relief of pain	33 patients
95%	Relief of pain	6 patients
90%	Relief of pain	17 patients
85%	Relief of pain	6 patients
80%	Relief of pain	11 patients
75%	Relief of pain	4 patients
70%	Relief of pain	9 patients
65%	Relief of pain	4 patients
60%	Relief of pain	3 patients
50%	Relief of pain	7 patients
40%	Relief of pain	1 patients
35%	Relief of pain	1 patients
0%	No benefit	2 patients

Location and type of pain treated

45 back	2 migraines
17 headache	2 feet
13 neck	1 tailbone
7 leg	1 elbow
5 shoulder	1 shingles
4 knee	1 stomach
4 hip	1 hand

surgeon Robert Becker makes a good case for nonunion fractures failing to mend because of an absence of electrical signals in the bone.[2] Is it too much of a stretch to think that diminished electrical activity may cause the degeneration of bone and other body parts, organs, or functions?

A case that makes me think broken Chi causes deterioration of the bone is the story of a nursing professor who came to me with severe knee pain. She had undergone seven knee surgeries three years earlier and now could not walk without crutches or a cane. She was told that a total knee replacement was her only hope, because the knee joint was so far gone. Three treatments stopped the pain for a year. Then she received two more treatments about a year apart when the pain began to return. Three more years have passed without a treatment and without severe pain in the knee. Now, with some arthritis in all of her joints, she feels the knee is the best joint in her body. A knee replacement is not even under consideration.

When Bioelectric and Auricular Therapy Do Not Work

Do the treatments help everyone? No. I know of at least three patients who took their lives because neither I nor anyone else could help them. Why the treatment does not help everyone with chronic pain is a question not fully understood. Below are some of the reasons we have discovered.

A patient came to me for pain that began after surgery. He was taking between twelve and twenty strong prescription painkillers a day, and had lost the function of his legs (because of the medication?). His electrical circuits were so shut off by the drugs that it was nearly impossible to turn them back on. He continued on the pain medication, stating that the doctor would not give it to him if it was harmful. The patient then went to the hospital to demand more medication and passed away. Although the pain medication may not have caused him to die, it is true that enough pain medication can cause respiratory arrest and death. Pain medication works against connecting the broken circuits and may block the results.

Caffeine and methyl xanthene medications were shown in a double-blind placebo study to block the analgesic effect of transcutaneous electric nerve stimulation (TENS). The amount of caffeine in just two or three cups of coffee makes TENS ineffective.[3]

Caffeine may also limit the effectiveness of Bioelectric and Auricular Therapy. One reason for this is that caffeine is a diuretic; it causes dehydration. Dehydration causes the body's electrical functions to fail. Electricity will not travel through dry tissue.

Infections the immune system does not or cannot deal with may limit the effectiveness of Bioelectric or Auricular treatments. The most dramatic healing I have ever seen came only after extracting a tooth with a root canal. Root canals can cause a myriad of inexplicable health problems, even when the teeth themselves appear healthy. (If you want to solve some of the most difficult and common health problems, read *A Healing Miracle* at *http:// www.healpain.net* or *Root Canal Cover-Up*, by George Meanig DDS.[4]) Patients with root canals can still be helped. Karen A., a young mother, came to me after spending over $100,000 trying to find relief from migraine headaches, chronic TMJ and neck pain. Three surgeries on her jaw, several root canals, caps, bridges, splints, and dental procedures too numerous to mention had left

Karen with a mouth that would not open straight and then only with pain. Oral surgeons and neurologists had run all of the tests and told her in so many words that the mechanics of her jaw were now perfect, so her pain must be psychological.

With the first treatment, Karen's jaw popped open and her eyes grew large. The pain was gone. With three more treatments, she felt she was completely healed and came back six months later to prove it to me. Since then, the condition has returned twice, but each time one treatment has brought total relief. Because Karen has had multiple root canals, she may never completely recover, but almost total relief for extended periods is available to her.

A patient named Que Barton asked if he would be able to play the piano after the treatment. I explained that the treatment was noninvasive, that we used only millionths of an amp (current too low even to be felt), and that the tiny seeds on his ear would certainly not have any bearing on his being able to play the piano. I told him, "When you don't hurt, you should be able to play even better," wherein he replied, "That's wonderful! Because I couldn't play the piano before the treatment."

Has Electrical Stimulation Been Proven?

Because I have suggested that electrical stimulation may help pain, medical professionals may recall a controlled study in the June 7, 1990 *New England Journal of*

Medicine (p.1627) that concluded, " . . . for patients with chronic low back pain, treatment with TENS is no more effective than treatment with a placebo, and TENS adds no apparent benefit to that of exercise alone." What this study really showed was how little the authors knew about electricity and its effect on the body. The researchers, like the FDA, assumed that all TENS are the same. This would be like saying, "We tried a drug in a controlled study that was found to be ineffective" and concluding that *all drugs* are no better than placebos.

There are endless combinations of waveforms, frequencies, harmonic frequencies, intensities, and methods as to how and where the stimulus is applied in electrical stimulation. To say that one is not effective does not tell you anything about the others any more than testing one drug tells you about all drugs.

With the correct, biologically compatible current properly applied, it often takes about twelve seconds to turn a body circuit on and thus stop pain. TENS pads stimulate five times too much per minute, three hundred times too much per hour. Implanted electrical devices for back pain, which cannot be moved, over-stimulate by a factor of thousands, not to mention the circuits they miss.

Summary on Treating Pain

If the ultimate cause of pain is the cutting, breaking, or suppression of the body's electrical circuits, what causes the circuits to fail when there is no injury, infection, tumor, or underlying pathology? Seven-time Nobel

Prize nominee and biochemist Joanna Budwig states that the electron flow across cell membranes and cell respiration is blocked by the "suffocating presence of saturated fats and hardened vegetable oils" (all margarine and all shortening, no matter what they are made of). Such "trans fatty acids" or hydrogenated vegetable oils may not only be a contributing factor to heart disease and cancer, but may be implicated in various pain syndromes as well.

Chronic dehydration also causes the body's electrical functions to fail. As we age, our thirst mechanism fails. We begin to fail to discern our own need to drink water, and most of us have dry joints, dry cartilage, dry tendons, and dry muscles—all of which can cause pain, because electricity will not travel through dry (dehydrated) tissue.

The success in treating patients on diuretics is limited because of water loss. I believe the number one cause of non-injury pain is dehydration. Drinking more water will cure most pain. This is discussed further in Chapter Four.

Another reason for the failure of our body's electrical functions can be illustrated with simple chemistry. Distilled water will not conduct electricity, and reverse osmosis-treated water is a poor conductor. If you add minerals to your water, or drink water that has not been distilled or been through reverse osmosis, the water becomes a better conductor. Biological cells lacking essential minerals will not conduct the electrical signals requisite to the pain-free functioning of a healthy body.

We have discovered some of the mysteries of this wonderful organism we call our body and what goes wrong when we hurt, but asking what shuts off the electrical circuits when there has been no accident or surgery may be as elusive as asking why electricity stops going across the brain when we die. If we discover the full answer to that question, we will have the "Methuselah pill."

We need pain to detect tumors, fractures, and ulcers, and to tell us when we are injured. We also need to know how to help those who hurt when pain is the disease, not the symptom. If the Bioelectric or Auricular therapeutic treatments are so effective, though, isn't there a danger of masking a serious underlying pathology of which pain is a symptom? There is less danger of covering up a serious medical condition with Bioelectric and Auricular therapy than there is when using pain medication, because the treatment will not work if the pain is being caused by a tumor, ulcer, bone fracture, or other pathology shutting off the body's electrical circuits and causing the pain. Auricular therapy reduces pain by correcting pain's cause, not by suppressing the pain signal.

After all that has been said about stopping pain, there are important lessons to be learned from pain. The following lines came to me in answer to the question of why we have pain:

We can remove the thorns from the roses
But even God will not spare us all pain.
For there is no joy without sorrow.
There can be no flowers without rain.

Notes

1. Nordenstrom, Bjorn, M.D., "Biologically Closed Electrical Circuits", *Nordic Medical Publications*, 1983.

2. Becker, Robert, M.D., *The Body Electric*, Morrow, 1987.

3. Marchand, Li, Charest, "Effects of Caffeine on Analgesia From Transcutaneous Electrical Nerve Stimulation", *New England Journal of Medicine*, Aug. 3, 1995, Vol. 333, No. 5, pp.325-326.

4. George Meanig D.D.S., "Root Canal Cover-Up," Available in the U.S. for $22.45 (includes shipping) from Bion Publishing, 323 E. Matilija 110-151, SD, Ojai CA 93023.

——

CHAPTER TWO

Why Surgery and Medication Are *Not* the Best Answers for Pain

*"The purpose of education is to replace
an empty mind with an open one."*
—Malcolm Forbes

ABSTRACT

$3.3 Billion Each Year Wasted on Useless Knee Surgery. Preventing Knee Pain. Surgery for Low Back Pain. Preventing Low Back and Leg Pain. Pain Medication (Non-Steroidal Anti-Inflammatory Drugs [NSAIDs]). Is Tylenol™ the Answer For Pain? Steroids (Cortisone) for Pain. Opioids (Narcotics) for Pain (codeine, oxycontin, fentanyl, hydrocodone, morphine, et al.). Is There a Better Way?

$3.3 Billion Each Year Wasted on Useless Knee Surgery

It is imperative to know the following about knee pain: The Houston Veterans Affairs Medical Center, Baylor College of Medicine, Houston, TX, conducted a randomized, placebo-controlled study of 180 patients to evaluate the efficacy of arthroscopic surgery for osteoarthritis of the knee. Conclusions: In this controlled trial involving patients with osteoarthritis of the knee, the outcomes after arthroscopic lavage or arthroscopic debridement were *no better* than those after a placebo procedure.[1]

Arthroscopic surgery for pain and knee stiffness caused by osteoarthritis is performed on about 650,000 people in the U.S. every year, at a cost of about $5,000 per procedure, for a total cost of $3.3 billion. And such surgery has been found to be no better than placebo surgery! (Note: The above information applies only to knee surgery for *osteoarthritis*, *not* knee surgery for any other reason.)

Preventing Knee Pain

103-year-old Larry Lewis jogged three miles every morning before going to work. He was the star of an educational motion picture that we made with Kenneth Cooper, who was the author of *Aerobics*. I had seen Larry Lewis in the film but did not meet him in person until I went to San Francisco to hold a California premier for the film at the St. Francis Hotel where Larry worked.

I arrived a day early to watch Larry at work before meeting him. I expected to see a elderly waiter pouring coffee or tea for the guests. Instead, I saw an incredibly vigorous old man running with large trays of food and carrying fifty-pound bags of flour on his shoulder to the kitchen. I then spent three days trying to keep up with the legendary Larry Lewis. After three days I decided that at 103 years of age, his heart must be in better shape than my heart at thirty-eight. I resolved to start jogging. "If he can do it, I can do it," I said.

Thirty years later, I'm still jogging regularly. My first three years of jogging, however, were hell because of the pain in my knees. Each morning I had to jog slowly for a mile or so before I could begin to run. I thought, "I have an old man's knees. Then I read an article in a medical journal explaining the cause of much of the knee pain people experience. What a discovery! The article was written by a Swedish orthopedic surgeon, who wrote, "One of the worst things you can do to your knees is crossing your legs." By this, he meant crossing your legs the way a man does, placing the outside of one ankle on top of the other knee and then letting the foreleg come down parallel to the ground. You know, the way cowboys cross their legs.

Crossing your legs the way a cowboy does torques the knee joint in a way that it is not supposed to bend. There is a lot of leverage between the ankle and the knee when the legs are crossed, especially if you have long legs. The leverage forces the joint in an unnatural way, causing chronic knee pain. I will not even show someone the wrong way to cross their legs, because if I do, my knees will hurt for three days when I run. My running is so important that I'll give $1,000 dollars to anyone who ever sees me cross my legs like a cowboy. I've been running regularly *without knee pain* for twenty-seven years because I never cross my legs the wrong way.

To have pain-free knees, there is something else people should know, especially athletes who suffer knee pain or who have sustained knee injuries: Never bend the knees below ninety degrees with weight on them. In other words, no *deep* knee bends. "Deep knee bends" is an exercise all football players had to do years ago. We have since learned that that deep knee bends stretch the tendons (which support the knee joint) too much and thus weaken the knee. When football players stopped having to do deep knee bends, football-related knee injuries were reduced by sixty percent. Nearly all football coaches now know this, even down to the junior high and high school levels. Doing "squats" with weights or knee bends down to ninety degrees is a good exercise to strengthen the knees, as long as you don't go further than keeping your upper legs parallel to the ground.

Another thing people need to do to prevent knee pain is to never wear shoes with heels that are "run over" (worn down on the outside edge). This stresses the knee joint because it throws the knee out of vertical alignment with the heel. Run over heels is one of the causes of chronic knee pain.

Surgery for Low Back Pain

The U.S. Department of Health and Human Services, Public Health Service commissioned the largest study of low back pain ever conducted at the beginning of the 1990s. It is titled "Understanding Acute Low Back Problems, Clinical Practice Guideline #14." A non-federal panel of experts sponsored by the Agency for Health Care Policy and Research (AHCPR) examined more than 3,900 scientific studies concerning the diagnosis and treatment of acute low back pain. The panel was consisted of twenty-three members—medical doctors, chiropractic doctors, nurses, experts in spinal research, physical therapists, an occupational therapist, a psychologist, and a consumer representative. Below are the exact words of one of their conclusions:

"Even having a lot of back pain does not by itself mean you need surgery. Surgery has been found to be helpful in only 1 in 100 cases of low back problems. In some people, surgery can even cause more problems. This is especially true if your only symptom is back pain."[2]

Acute pain will heal itself; chronic pain does not. If surgery will help only one in one hundred patients with acute low back pain, would the odds be any better for chronic back pain, which is even more resistant to healing?

Back pain is not mechanical. According to Lloyd Saberski, editor of *The Pain Clinic Journal*, "Pain is an electrochemical event and will not appear on an X-ray or MRI." Recently, a study by Dickey indicated that the mathematical possibility of predicting chronic pain based on imaging alone was 1:64,000. But what is the first thing most doctors do when you have unresolved back pain? Send you for an X-ray, CT scan, or MRI.

Unless a nerve is severed, it can function perfectly. The compression or pinching of a nerve causes pain or loss of function only if the signal going through the nerve is suppressed. Even with a pinched nerve, if the *signal* is not suppressed, a person can remain pain-free. What determines whether or not a person with a pinched nerve experiences pain is the signal traveling through the nerve, not the compression. Pinched nerves do not necessarily cause pain. Shut off or "broken" nerves are the cause of pain—whether or not the nerve is compressed.

"Surgical successes unfortunately only apply to approximately one percent of patients with low back pain." According to Alf Nachemson, M.D., editor of the journal *Spine,* bulging discs are found and taken as an excuse to do a lot of surgery and percutaneous discectomy. Discs are made to bulge; that is a normal finding."

Approximately 200,000 Americans undergo an initial spine surgery for the treatment of chronic low back pain annually according to a 1998 survey of spine surgeons. The same research indicates that about twenty-five percent (50,000) of these patients continue to experience unresolved pain after surgery. And, despite a second procedure to relieve the pain, more than thirteen thousand patients still suffer from unresolved pain.[3]

I have treated more than three thousand patients with low back pain, close to half of whom have had spinal surgery. When I ask those who have had back surgery whether they would do it again, if they had the chance to do so, most of them respond, "No, never again. I would never have the surgery!" Others answer, "Yes, because I had no choice. I would have been paralyzed if I hadn't had the surgery." In most cases I doubt this is true.

A doctor in Las Vegas, Nevada, who claims to have treated more than 21,000 patients with low back pain, states that other than accident victims, he has never seen a patient who became paralyzed by avoiding the recommended surgery. Rather, he has seen many people become paralyzed *after* having the spinal surgery. Of course, when the spinal cord or nerves are severed in an accident, anyone can become paralyzed.

The question is, how often do herniated disks, stenosis, or degenerative disk disease paralyze anyone? It is, of course, possible to lose function from a pinched nerve, but taking heavy pain medication may also shut off a nerve signal completely and cause loss of function. Do herniated disks without pain medication ever lead to paralysis? Conceivably, they could, but not as often as surgeons would like us to believe.

"Young man, you will be paralyzed in two months if you don't have surgery!" These words were spoken by a renowned spine surgeon to the son of a woman who worked in our clinic. Travis was scheduled for back surgery. While awaiting an appointment with the surgeon, he had the opportunity to overhear other patients in the waiting room. From their conversations he became aware of the fact that some of the patients were still in considerable pain after having had spinal surgery.

When Travis' turn came to see the doctor, being a brash young man, he asked the big question. "I've been out in your waiting room listening to some of the other patients. Some of them have already had surgery and are still in pain. Are you sure the operation is going to help me?" The surgeon pointed his finger at Travis and said, "Young man, you will be paralyzed in two months if you don't have surgery!" I treated Travis. After one treatment he was pain-free for three years. I then treated him again. That treatment was also successful. Now six years later, although Travis is troubled with recurrent low back pain, he is not paralyzed.

Another young man was scheduled for back surgery, and about a week before he was to have it, his pain completely disappeared. When he reported this to the surgeon and asked whether he still needed surgery, the surgeon replied, "Oh, absolutely. You might sneeze and become totally paralyzed!" With such a prognosis from such a famous doctor, the surgery was performed. After the surgery, the man realized his mistake, because he now had different and even more severe pain than he had before surgery.

Another case shows how bizarre back surgery experiences can be. I treated a man in Idaho Falls. The following Monday morning when I arrived at my office, his brother-in-law from Northern California was waiting for me. He had gone to a neurosurgeon with low back pain. The surgeon ordered an MRI spine scan. After reading the scan, the surgeon said, "We can't see anything wrong with your lower back, but the disk spaces in your *neck* are severely narrowed. That's where the problem is!" Surgery was performed on his cervical vertebra and he was presented with a bill for $60,000. But the surgery did nothing for the lower back pain. Rather, it created a new pain, in the man's neck, a place he had never experienced pain before.

My opinion of spinal surgery is no doubt distorted because I see only patients whose surgeries were unsuccessful, but I am not alone in my opinion. Unsuccessful back surgery is not uncommon. There is even a special name for patients who experience such an outcome: "Failed Spine Surgery Syndrome," or FSSS. I see many patients who hurt more after spinal surgery than before they had it, and I would like to see someone do a randomized, placebo-controlled study on spinal surgery similar to the study done on surgery for osteoarthritis knee pain.

I believe the placebo or sham surgery might prove to be as effective for reducing pain as the real surgery. I also believe that, other than for severed nerves and fractured bones, the only terms under which spinal surgery should be performed to cure pain is, "If the surgery doesn't reduce the pain, or if it makes it worse, the surgeon shouldn't be paid." I don't think you would find a surgeon in the U.S. who would operate under those terms.

Most spinal surgeons, to their credit, do not tell patients that they will be paralyzed if they do not have surgery. Rather, they advise against surgery, saying, "When the pain gets so bad that you can't stand it any longer, we will operate. Until then, I will not operate." When a patient begs for surgery, if it fails, the surgeon is off the hook.

Circumstances in which spinal decompression surgery is considered imperative includes muscle wasting, loss of bowel or kidney control and loss of motor function. Even with these symptoms, I believe the patient can still be helped if you can increase the signal going through the compressed nerve (which is what I do). This is probably beyond what any spinal surgeon considers possible. It is also beyond what chiropractors claim to do. When a chiropractor makes his adjustment to correct a "subluxation" or pinched nerve, he must then depend on the body to increase the signal going through the nerve. This may or may not happen. That is why you have to go back to the chiropractor so many times.

Because most spinal surgeries are not done for muscle wasting, loss of bowel or kidney control, or loss of motor function, I offer a challenge: Send me ten or more patients who are scheduled for back surgery and I'll guarantee to stop the pain with one or two treatments (usually one) in more than half of the patients—because I will correct what causes the pain, not simply cover it up, even if the nerve is compressed.

I make the above challenge with the qualification that the patients must be hydrated and not taking heavy pain medication. I prefer that they are taking no pain medication. My work is to repair or connect broken or impaired neurological signals. Pain medication shuts the signals off.

A procedure that truly addresses the cause of pain will help patients on the first treatment. Any health care practitioner who keeps the patient coming back again and again, in my mind, is suspect. You don't know whether the treatment is helping or if the body is healing itself over time. A doctor once told me that his professors in medical school had told him, "Patients would come back every week of their lives whether they needed to or not if the doctor told them to do so." The doctor added, "I didn't believe it at the time, but it's true!" And that's the way he practices. To each patient he says, "I want to see you again in a week," "I want to see you in two weeks," or "I want to see you again in a month." He has one of the largest practices in the state.

If you call a plumber and he doesn't fix your leak, he doesn't get paid. If he tries again and again fails to fix the leak, should he get paid twice? The same is true of an auto mechanic. If he doesn't fix your car, he doesn't get paid. Should medical and health care professionals be any less accountable?

Paying doctors for thousands of surgeries that are no more effective than placebos, and paying health care providers for endless treatments patients don't need (whether the cost is paid by the patient or the insurance company), are practices that must change. Correcting the system can begin with you.

Preventing Low Back and Leg Pain

There is a simple exercise you can do (even in bed) to *prevent* most low back pain. While lying on your back, cross your arms and put each hand on the opposite shoulder. Then with your knees bent, do sit ups. Start with just one or two sit-ups and work up to ten sit-ups a day. If you do a minimum of ten sit ups every day religiously, and if you are not dehydrated, it will prevent nearly all low back pain, except for the kind of low back pain that travels directly down the hamstring or the very back of the leg.

Regular stretching of the hamstring can prevent the kind of low back pain that radiates down the very back of the leg. Exercise and aging cause the hamstrings and heel cords to shorten and tighten. When the hamstrings shorten, it can pull tissue away from the spine and lower back, causing extreme low back pain. When the heel cords shorten, they pull tissue away from the bone, causing pain in the lower part of the leg or knee. Proper and regular (daily) stretching will prevent low back pain that radiates down the very back of the leg and pain in the lower leg.

The best way to stretch tight hamstrings is to sit on the edge of a bed or couch and put one leg up to the side on the bed or couch, then *gently* straighten that leg. You will feel it pull the hamstring tight as you straighten the leg. Take several days, even weeks, to lengthen the hamstrings.

Stretching the hamstrings too tightly or too quickly could pull tissue away from the lower back, causing severe low back pain. When stretching the hamstrings, it is ideal to hold *gentle* pressure on the hamstring for several minutes. You could do this every night, even while watching TV.

Once the hamstrings are stretched, you will not need to do the stretching exercise as long or as often. A habit of doing at least some stretching every day will keep the hamstrings from becoming shorter and tighter and will ultimately prevent the low back pain that radiates down the back of the leg.

If you have pain in the lower leg and/ or shin splints, an effective way to stretch heel cords is to stand facing a wall. Place your hands on the wall, and, keeping your hands on the wall, slowly back away from the wall with your feet until you feel your heel cords *gently* pulled tight. Hold the position for about 10-25 seconds. Do this exercise at least once a day.

Another exercise to stretch heel cords is to stand on something that slants uphill, or to pull the toes and front of the foot up. Some people even make a slant board to stand on when they work at a counter or wash dishes. If you have chronic pain in the lower leg, you may need to repeat the exercises several times a day. *The stretching should be gentle.* Pulling the heel cords too tight or stretching them too quickly could cause shin splints or lower leg pain instead of preventing them.

One must *never* exercise or do physical labor when dehydrated. We've all heard the following advice to prevent back injuries from hundreds of sources: Keep your back straight when lifting. Keep all lifted objects close to your body. Lift with your leg muscles. Avoid lifting while twisting, bending forward, reaching, etc. Far, far more important than any of these is that you never lift, stretch, or exercise when you are dehydrated.

It is when you are dehydrated that you "pull" muscles and break the body's endogenous electrical connections between cells. Again, this causes pain. So often when someone has their "back go out," it is *not* from heavy lifting but from bending or twisting to pick up a piece of paper or other small object. Those kinds of injuries occur when you are dehydrated. The injury would not have happened if the person was properly hydrated. If athletes would drink twice as much water as they think they need before competing, it would reduce athletic injuries immeasurably.

It is important that you not do the "in-bed sit-ups" or stretching exercises first thing in the morning before drinking water. Unless you drink water during the night, you will be dehydrated when you first wake up. Everyone is dehydrated in the morning because we lose 2-4 pounds of water vapor through respiration while we sleep. You can prove that to yourself by weighing carefully when you go to bed and again in the morning when upon awakening. You will find that you are 2-4 pounds lighter in the morning, even if you haven't urinated during the night.

Electrical signals will not travel through dry tissue. This is why many people hurt worse when they first get up in the morning; the electrical signals connecting the cells are impaired. If the signals fail because of dehydration, you can hurt just as much as if you had been hit by a hammer. You may want to keep water next to the bed and drink it before rising. Then you should wait twenty minutes or so before exercising or stretching.

Pain Medication
(Non-Steroidal Anti-Inflammatory Drugs [NSAIDs])

Traditional Western medicine offers two options for pain: surgery and/ or drugs. Are pain medications harmless—even as they stop the pain? All over-the-counter medications (except for acetaminophen) and some prescription medications for pain are known as non-steroidal anti-inflammatory drugs (NSAIDs). These include aspirin, ibuprofen, indomethacin, naproxen, oxaprozin, piroxicam, sulindac, and more than twelve others. All of them may cause gastrointestinal bleeding.

Bleeding from taking NSAIDs is no small problem. A study published in *JAMA* 279.1200-1205, appearing in

1998, estimated that seventy-six thousand persons in the U.S. were hospitalized in 1994 because of taking NSAIDs, mostly because of gastrointestinal bleeding. Approximately ten percent of those hospitalized died. That's seventy-six thousand people who die unnecessarily every year from taking anti-inflammatory pain medication! (This does not include the unknown numbers of people who die from internal bleeding who were *not* hospitalized.) Known deaths from taking NSAIDs kills twice as many people every year as were killed in the attack on the World Trade Centers. Is anyone making war on NSAIDs?

A recent study published in *The Archives of Internal Medicine,* June 2000, 160: 777-784, found that NSAIDs caused a greater than tenfold increase in the risk of congestive heart failure (CHF) in patients with a history of heart disease. In those without a history of heart disease, the use of NSAIDs still increased the risk by sixty percent.

Is Tylenol™ the Answer for Pain?

Tylenol™ (acetaminophen), with sales well over one billion dollars a year, is the best-selling over-the-counter pain medication. It is neither an anti-inflammatory nor a steroid. Unlike NSAIDs, Tylenol™ does *not* cause gastrointestinal bleeding. But is it completely safe? The makers of Tylenol™ would like you to believe so, when taken at the recommended doses. But what is the truth? And what are the possible side effects of acetaminophen use?

"New Painkiller Labels Just for Kids." This was the large headline on a 1997 *Associated Press* news release. The article stated, "Relatively small overdoses of acetaminophen—Tylenol's™ active ingredient—have been blamed for liver damage and even death in children in the United States."

The *Journal of Pediatrics,* January, 1998, p. 132, reported the following: At least twenty-four children in the United States have died and three have required liver transplants after receiving accidental overdoses of acetaminophen—the most widely used medication for relief of pain and fever in children and infants. Researchers say parents should be advised about the dangers of exceeding the recommended doses of the drug, which are based on the child's body weight. The report is a compilation of fifty-five documented cases of accidental liver toxicity in children attributed to acetaminophen given in doses above those recommended. Of the two dozen deaths, six were due to multiple acetaminophen doses only slightly above weight-based recommendations. (Note the phrase, "*slightly above.*")

"No other over-the-counter drug has a narrower range between therapy and toxicity than acetaminophen," says Dr. William Lee, a recognized expert on liver disease and professor of internal medicine at the University of Texas' Southwestern Medical Center in Dallas. Dr. Lee and colleagues followed 295 patients who had liver failure. Acetaminophen overdose was the most common identified cause, affecting sixty patients, or twenty percent of the group. According to Dr. Lee, acetaminophen appears to be the single leading cause of acute liver failure.

Because acetaminophen is found in almost two hundred different products, taking a few different remedies on the same day can unknowingly lead to toxic doses. An FDA review found more than fifty-six thousand emergency room visits a year due to acetaminophen overdoses, about a quarter of them unintentional.

Both the *New England Journal of Medicine* and the *Journal of the American Medical Association* published articles advising against using acetaminophen if you consume alcoholic beverages. Why is this a potentially deadly combination? Because both are harmful to the liver.

Pronouncements from Johnson & Johnson, makers of Tylenol™, proclaim Tylenol™ to be absolutely safe at the recommended dose. However, as far as I know, no one has ever done a study on the long-term cumulative effects of regular acetaminophen use in human populations. I suspect long-term use of acetaminophen would take its toll on the liver the way alcohol does. Others believe the same. Although never implemented, in 1977, FDA advisors recommended that we not take acetaminophen for more than ten days "because severe liver damage may occur."

Even though hospitals in the U.S. are not required to report cases, acetaminophen, alone and in combination with other products, was the leading cause of accidental and suicidal drug fatalities reported to poison control centers in 1996. In second place were cocaine drug fatalities, which were twenty-five percent lower than acetaminophen fatalities.

As of September 2002, a warning has appeared on Tylenol™ labels regarding alcohol consumption and a statement that overdoses in children "could cause serious health problems." On a large package of Extra Strength Tylenol™, there is a warning that if children accidentally overdose on Tylenol™, "Call a poison control center immediately, whether there are any symptoms or not." Nothing is said about possible liver failure and/ or death from overdose.

When taken over extended periods of time, acetaminophen can also cause permanent kidney damage. This damage can be lethal to those with underlying kidney disease. One study showed that people who used acetaminophen with other pain relievers on a regular basis had a three to eightfold increase in their risk of kidney cancer. Joseph Mercola M.D. claims that about fifteen percent of people on dialysis today are there as a result of the damage that Tylenol™ and/ or aspirin did to their kidneys.

Why not inform those who use acetaminophen about possible kidney damage or liver failure? Johnson & Johnson says that "organ specific" warnings would confuse people. Why doesn't the warning say anything about the risk of death from overdose? That would promote suicides, the company says. If people knew that overdoses of acetaminophen were potentially deadly, they might use Tylenol™ to take their lives. Apparently, J&J is more concerned about causing the death of someone who wants to die than about preventing the death of someone who wants to feel better.

Laws to prevent intentional overdoses limits the amount of acetaminophen you can buy at one time in England. Because of what has become somewhat common knowledge in Great Britain, people don't need doctors such as Kevorkian to help them end their lives.

For more information about acetaminophen warnings, deaths, and out-of-court settlements paid to plaintiffs under agreements that require them to keep mum about the terms, see: *Forbes* January 12, 1998 article "J&J's Dirty Little Secret."[4] The last sentences of the above article from *Forbes* reads, "Ralph Larsen (J&J's CEO) has a painful choice. He can rewrite the label, putting on it the verbal equivalent of a skull and crossbones. Or he can go on paying off victims, and hope for the best. Which is the moral choice? Which, in the long run, is the best business decision?"

The inexorable law of marketing is, "When a product is no longer profitable, it will no longer be sold." Acetaminophen, aluminum antiperspirants, amalgam tooth fillings, local anesthetics, NSAIDs, root canals, and X-rays will go the way of Fen-phen, Premarin, and arthroscopic knee surgery for osteoarthritis. I don't think any of them will give up as quietly as Mercurochrome or Merthiolate. More likely, each will go the way of cigarettes, kicking and screaming like Virginia Slim, the Marlboro man, and Joe Camel. Until then, there are not millions, but billions, of dollars to be made. Advertising has misled thousands of doctors and millions of patients into thinking that all of the above products and procedures (acetaminophen to X-rays) are not harmful.

Another reason given for not putting stronger warnings on Tylenol™ is that people would switch to NSAIDs (most certainly true), which cause gastrointestinal bleeding. Is either one a good choice? Would you prefer potential death from gastrointestinal bleeding and congestive heart failure, or from liver or kidney failure? The other options are steroids and narcotics.

Steroids (Cortisone) for Pain

"Cortisone shots are the thing for athletic injuries, because they are fast, they are easy, and they work." These words were spoken by an orthopedic surgeon. He then added that he "would inject a site up to three times a year but no more, because more than that risks tendon rupture."

Injected cortisone dissolves muscle, tendons, ligaments, cartilage, bone, and nerves. It stops pain by destroying the nerve. This means the pain signal cannot get through to the brain. Then when the nerve tries to heal or reconnect, the pain returns, often worse than ever.

What the surgeon above was really saying is, "I'm going to dissolve the muscle, tendons, ligaments, cartilage bone, and nerves, right to the point where the tendons will snap in two, and that is okay because it's quick, it's easy, and it works."

Athletes are injected with cortisone when they are injured, then sent back into the game. When they become invalids and lose function because of the damage done by the cortisone, they blame the athletics.

A friend of mine, who is a professor of physical education, received numerous cortisone injections for "tennis elbow." The tendons ruptured and he lost partial use of his arm. Don't tell him, "Cortisone shots are the thing for athletic injuries, because they are fast, they are easy, and they work."

Opioids (Narcotics) for Pain (codeine, oxycontin, fentanyl, hydrocodone, morphine, et al.)

"No one needs to have pain. If you have pain it is because you are not taking enough medication or because you are not taking the right medication for you." These were the words of a prominent anesthesiologist, trained at the Mayo Clinic, speaking to an auditorium filled with people who had come to attend a seminar on pain.

The other point this doctor stressed was, "You don't have to worry about addiction when you are giving narcotics for severe pain. People do not become addicted after the need for the medication has ended."

Addiction is *not* the problem. How would taking pain medication the rest of your life be any different than taking insulin or high blood pressure medication the rest of your life? Instead of addiction, the problem is all the other harmful side effects narcotics present, which the doctor did not mention. Paralyzed bowels, for example. Narcotics are well known for causing constipation. When that issue came up in the seminar, the doctor dismissed the problem with, "Then we just give the patient a stool softener."

I became aware of how pervasive narcotic-caused constipation is when I was called upon to help relieve the suffering of a terminal cancer patient who had been sent home to die. I saw the patient after fourteen days of morphine treatment for pain. On the fourteenth day, the patient was delirious. I consulted with a trusted doctor, who said, "If his bowels do not move before morning, you will bury him." The patient, who had not had a bowel movement in five days, died the next morning.

When the patient was autopsied, his bowels were *empty*. The body was trying so desperately to heal the cancer that it reabsorbed all the feces from the bowels that were paralyzed by morphine. Although I could not say this then to his family, this is what caused the delirium. This is what killed the patient, not the cancer.

I wonder how many terminal cancer patients die from paralyzed bowels caused by taking morphine, even though cancer is the reported cause of death.

Concern for addiction is not an issue when giving opioids to terminal cancer patients. It may not be a major problem when given for severe, intractable pain. But the possibility of abuse by others who get their hands on the drugs is overwhelming.

A recent television special showed the magnitude of OxyContin™ (oxycodone) abuse, particularly in West Virginia. It is spreading rapidly to other states. Law enforcement officials expressed the opinion that OxyContin™ is more addicting than heroin. It seems that every family in the state of West Virginia has been negatively impacted by OxyContin™ abuse—either by having their drug stolen by an addict, having a family member become addicted, having a family member die from an overdose of it, or having a family member murdered.

On the other side of the abuse issue is an unending lobby of people with intractable pain who are demanding access to OxyContin™ and other narcotics. Their pain is so severe that many say they will take their lives if they are denied what they believe are life-saving drugs—drugs abusers will kill to get.

It is not the purpose of this paper to list all of the harmful side effects of pain medication. The harmful, life-altering, life-destroying side effects and abuse of opioids and other pain medications are too numerous to mention. More important than listing the side effects is to reveal a better way to treat pain.

If you want to know the harmful effects of the pain medication you are taking, read the warnings (small print) on over-the-counter medications. To the credit of many NSAID manufacturers, the warnings say, "May cause serious bleeding and even *death*."

For prescription medications, ask your pharmacist for the leaflet that gives the precautions, warnings, and counter indications. When you do this, you will realize that all prescription medications (for anything, not just pain) are a contradiction of the Hippocratic Oath, which is: "First Do No Harm." Only the doctor is supposed to know if the potential benefits of taking a prescription are greater than the potential harm. The possibility of a medication being injurious exists with every prescription medication. That's why they are controlled substances.

Is There a Better Way?

It is the philosophy, approach, and very foundation of those interested in pain management to suppress the pain signal or alter the perception of pain in the brain. That approach is fatally flawed. It never has and never will eliminate pain without side effects. You cannot suppress sensory nerves (the pain signal) without suppressing other vital functions—bowels, liver, kidney, respiratory, motor, or mental. Suppressing the pain signal is harmful to the body no matter how you do it.

Treating pain can be compared to fighting a war. You can fight a war when you don't know exactly who the enemy is, but you can never win. That is why pain management spokespeople speak only of managing pain; you never hear them speak about healing pain.

Western doctors don't know exactly what pain is, so they attack the pain signal (symptom) with medication—medications that kill far more people each year than the attack on the World Trade Centers.

The enemy is not the pain signal, not the symptom, not the harmful medications, not the doctors who prescribe medication. The enemy in the war on pain is what causes the pain in the first place: broken electrical connections between cells. Treating the cause of the pain instead of the pain symptom itself is better. It is the only way to *heal* pain.

> *"God whispers to us in our pleasures,*
> *speaks to our conscience, but shouts*
> *in our pains."*
>
> —C. S. Lewis

Notes

1. For the full study see: *New England Journal of Medicine* 2002 Jul 11; 347(2): 81-8.

2. For more information about guidelines or to receive a free, printed copy of the consumer version of *Understanding Acute Low Back Problems,* call toll-free: (800) 358-9295, or write to: Agency for Health Care Policy and Research Publications Clearinghouse, P.O. Box 8547, Silver Spring, MD 20907.

3. For more information see: *http://www.nsnonline.org/FBSS/ pressrelease.html.*

4. For the *Forbes* full article see: *http://www.torahview.com/ bris/html/Tylenol™.html.*

———

CHAPTER THREE

The *Only* Way to Heal Pain

Connecting the "Broken Chi" that Causes Pain

*"You do not have to be a genius . . .
The major work of the world is done by
ordinary people who have learned to work
in an extraordinary way."*

—Gordon B. Hinckley

ABSTRACT

Pain Healed "Immediately" by Applying Biotape™, a Highly *Conductive*, Patented, Polymer Membrane. Treating Pain and Other Diseases with Scar Therapy, Prolotherapy and Biotape™. Banana Peels *Will* Stop Headaches, Ann Landers (the good doctor is wrong!). Conductive Headache Bands.

Pain Healed "Immediately" by Applying Biotape™, a Highly Conductive, Patented, Polymer Membrane.

The following is condensed from an article I wrote. It was published in the August/ September 1998 *Townsend Letter for Doctors* (note: the dates are relevant to that time):

This paper presents a method to verify (for the first time) with "double-blind" placebo controlled studies, the two thousand-year-old Chinese definition of pain. The Chinese believe that *pain* is caused by the "blockage of Chi"—a concept that has never been adequately evaluated in Western medicine. I submit that "Chi" is the endogenous electrical potential in living tissue that can be accurately measured and quantified. I further propose that pain is caused by cut, broken, or suppressed electrical connections between cells.

In support of the theory, and through my practice of auricular medicine, I have measured the electrical resistance at the site of pain in more than eighteen thousand treatments. Where there is pain, the electrical resistance is always high, indicating a blockage or suppression of the body's electrical signals.

To further evaluate the Chinese theory of pain, I developed a highly conductive, polymer membrane to be applied over the site of pain. Once the membrane is applied, it acts (electrically) like a living part of the body.

Below are case studies (from more than twelve hundred) in which the membrane was applied to relieve pain. The membrane (hereafter referred to by the trade name Biotape™) is chemically inert. No medicine, drugs, or external electricity is used with or applied by or through the tape.

Lois C.: Excruciating endless pain since knee surgery in 1987. Biotape™ applied 12-12-96. Patient reported eight months later that the relief of pain from one application of the tape "is the greatest joy in my entire life." After nine years of relentless pain, patient is still pain-free eight months after treatment.

Carolyn A.: Fibromyalgia. Disabling neck and shoulder pain for six years. Patient spent more than two hours every night hot-packing her shoulder just to be able to function as the breadwinner for her family. Biotape™ applied 4-22-97, providing seventy percent immediate relief. Reapplied tape 5-21-97. Patient reported two months later that her neck and shoulder were completely healed.

Marvin W.: Peripheral Neuropathy. Balls of feet almost too tender to walk on for five years. Biotape™ applied 7-7-97. "There was instant relief and no pain until the tape came off."

Mary E.: Sciatic pain. Biotape™ applied 6-18-97. Patient bent over immediately after and said, "That's the first time I have been able to bend over without pain in ten years!" Pain a month later still only about ten percent of what it was before treatment.

Tricia M.: Low back pain so severe she couldn't stand or walk. Used magnets (being touted for pain) for a week.

The magnets did not help (because magnets are not conductive). Biotape™ relieved pain immediately and patient could stand and walk.

Obviously not all cases are this successful, but they are representative of what does occur more often than could be attributed to a placebo. (**For more case studies on using Biotape for pain relief, see:** *http://www.healpain.net.* **New, fourth generation Biotape™, with a U.S. patent and skin-friendly adhesive is available for consumer use from Smart Inventions, Inc., 6319 E. Alondra Blvd., Paramount, CA 90723-3750. Call toll free, 1-800-977-6336.**) Note: No medical claims are made for Biotape™. The information above is only anecdotal until established by double-blind, placebo-controlled medical studies. Not all patients respond equally well or permanently.

The existence of endogenous electrical signals in the body is not in question. It is a measurable phenomenon. If electrical nerve signals are blocked, cells will die or degenerate, causing muscle wasting. All muscular movements are controlled by electricity. The heart works electrically. If the heart's sinus node fails, an electrical pacemaker is implanted. We are "brain dead" when there are no more electrical signals crossing the brain. Cell death occurs when there are no more electrical signals crossing the cell.

Western medicine primarily addresses the chemical and mechanical functions of the body. Traditional Chinese medicine deals with electrical processes. Acupuncture points cannot be seen, but they can be found with modern electronic instruments called "point finders." The points are areas of low electrical resistance and are no bigger than the head of a pin. Incredibly, acupuncture points are precisely where the Chinese have said they were for centuries!

Western medicine can name many conditions believed to cause pain. It is known in nanoseconds how fast pain signals travel to the brain. Science has discovered the pain control chemicals that the body produces in the brain and spinal column. Blocking the pain signal with drugs is a highly developed science. Still, Western medicine does not understand the physiology of pain or how to heal it. Pain is caused by injured tissue, but what causes pain when there has been no injury? How does the body heal pain?

Evidence that proves that Western medicine has not yet learned the cause of pain is its dependence on imaging devices such as X-rays, CT scans, and MRIs to reveal the cause of pain. Imaging instruments show only mechanical damage. They reveal nothing about soft tissue damage or about the body's electrical signals. Imaging devices cannot see endogenous electrical signals (Chi) in the body, and cannot reveal broken connections.

A study published in the *Mayo Clinic Proceedings* provides more such evidence.[1] The study reported that in ninety-four percent of cases, the search for the cause of chronic pain is unsuccessful. The essence of another monumental review of seven hundred published pain studies was that it is a waste of valuable resources to keep searching for the cause of chronic pain, because the cause of most instances of chronic pain cannot be discovered. Since the above studies were published, new drugs have been discovered, new and more sophisticated methods of delivering the drugs have been developed, and we are still left only with pain management—treating the symptom and not the cause. For this reason, in 2003, more than ninety percent of the time, modern medicine is still unsuccessful in discovering the cause of chronic pain.

Traditional Chinese medicine has understood what pain is for more than two thousand years. We now offer a simple method anyone can use to relieve pain or verify the Chinese definition of pain. Double-blind placebo-controlled studies could easily be done using the conductive tape and a non-conductive tape with an identical appearance. Neither the doctor nor the patient would know who is getting the real thing and who the placebo.

The reason we do not do our own double-blind study is because our outcome would be questioned. Such a study should be performed independently of the Pain Research Institute. We will provide materials and training to any independent researcher who has experience in conducting and has published double-blind studies. A positive outcome from such a study would be evidence for what is almost inconceivable, that Western medicine has never learned the cause of pain!

Treating Pain and Other Diseases with Scar Therapy, Prolotherapy, and Biotape™

Scar therapy and prolotherapy are two methods of treating pain and other health problems that hundreds of U.S. alternative, complementary, or integrative doctors, osteopaths, and health care practitioners are using with success.

Scar therapy is legendary for helping people with long-standing health problems of every kind where traditional medicine has failed. The process involves injecting small amounts of procaine every third or fourth of an inch down both sides of every scar on the body. The theory is that the scars or incision have disrupted energy fields in the body, which leads to bad health. Injecting procaine is supposed to reestablish the energy traveling across the scar. Does it work? It is very successful for some patients. Scar therapy is all some doctors do. Their fame has spread and, people with every imaginable malady and difficult health problem come to them from all over the world. It does help a percentage of them even with the most difficult problems.

Prolotherapy (also known as reconstructive or sclero-therapy) is the king of treatments for pain by alternative, complementary, and integrative medical practitioners. Prolotherapy (similar to scar therapy) consists of injecting small amounts of local anesthetics (procaine, lidocaine, xylocaine, etc.) and sugar water as a proliferant into trigger points associated with the pain instead of along scars or incisions. The injected dextrose acts as an irritant (proliferant), which causes inflammation that the body then theoretically heals, along with whatever was causing the pain in the first place. It is a means of treating pain by creating pain (irritation) with the injected dextrose advocates refer to as a "minor irritant."

Where scar therapy is for all health problems, Prolotherapy is generally only for pain. Prolotherapy is successful for most types pain. Pain clinics specializing in prolotherapy are springing up all over the country. One local doctor has been so successful in his application of prolotherapy that he has created a chain of such clinics.

You may have heard of GH-3 and Ana Aslan, the famous doctor in Romania to whom many celebrities went for anti-aging treatments. GH-3 is primarily injected procaine. Does procaine prevent aging? Thousands said it did, probably because the high they got from the procaine made them feel better. Chemically, procaine is a close relative of the street drug cocaine. Much scientific research conducted since Ana Aslan's application of procaine has shown that it has no effect on the aging process.

Now the bad news: Local anesthetics (procaine, lidocaine, xylocaine, etc.), when injected into the body, are converted to an aniline that is a known carcinogen (cancer-causing agent).

Alfred Nickel, an oral surgeon, provides the following information about injected anesthetics: "All local anesthetics currently approved for use in the United States (lidocaine, mepivacaine, bupivacaine, procaine, etc.) are broken down in the body to anilines. The FDA did studies to determine if the breakdown of local anesthetics to anilines is correct, and in 1993, demonstrated that human tissues exposed to lidocaine (the most commonly used local anesthetic) converted 67% of the lidocaine to a known aniline (2,6-xylidine). This particular aniline is a recognized animal and, very probably human carcinogen capable of causing breast cancer (animal studies 99.999% causative), prostate cancer, brain cancer, leukemia, sarcomas, carcinomas, and, in fact, pretty much the whole spectrum of recognized cancers. The aniline (2,6-xylidine) is one of the carcinogenic chemical components of tobacco, but we now know that *injecting 1 cc of 2% lidocaine will result in the same aniline dose as smoking 94,000 unfiltered cigarettes!*" [2]

In 1993, the FDA found the lowest dose tested of a metabolite from the topical anesthetic Emla caused cancer in both rats and mice. The *Biennial Report on Carcinogens* states that local anesthetics fulfill the requirements for listing as "reasonably anticipated to be a human carcinogen," and the FDA now requires a cancer warning in the package inserts of new pharmaceuticals containing aniline-based local anesthetics. (Why not require the warning on all local anesthetics and not just the new ones?)

When Dr. Nickel contacted the FDA about the need for warning labels, "The FDA insisted that, lacking alternative non-carcinogenic local anesthetics, regulation of these pharmaceuticals would be dependent on considerations of risk verses benefit." How can a doctor or dentist make that decision if he does not know the danger? Most doctors and dentists do not know the danger of local anesthetics.

Medical procedures and dentistry can be performed, and endured, without local anesthesia. (I will teach anyone interested how to do finger press anesthesia for dental procedures.) How much better it would be if the doctor knew and patients were given a choice of whether or not to receive local anesthetics (or X-rays) that may lead to cancer.

All cigarette advertisements in the U.S. include a warning that the cigarettes may cause cancer. Shouldn't all doctors' offices and clinics performing scar therapy, prolotherapy, or using local anesthetics have a warning sign on their front doors?

I have conducted more than eighteen thousand treatments without drugs or the painful injections required for scar therapy or prolotherapy. Scar therapy can be performed with Biotape™ simply by placing the tape across scars and incisions. I submit the following letter as evidence:

Dear Mr. Stoddard,

I wanted to let you know how much the Biotape™ treatment has improved my health. The improvement is remarkable. The pains in my arms have almost disappeared, and my energy level is up significantly. My overall health has definitely stepped up a level. I am so grateful for the help that you have given me.

My health has been deteriorating over the last twenty years. In the early 1980s I started experiencing allergy problems. In 1986, I began having bowel problems. The bowel and allergy problems continued through the 1990s. In 1998, after several high-stress life experiences, my health took an even more significant turn for the worse. At that time, my digestive system completely failed and I began experiencing heart palpitations, weakness in my body, and strange pains in my arms, back, and shoulders. I was so ill that I couldn't go to work for a month. After receiving little help from conventional medicine, I realized that conventional therapies weren't going to get me back on my feet.

I began exploring alternative therapies and lifestyles. I worked with numerous alternative therapists. I tried just about everything, including a special diet, mercury detoxification, green food, pro-biotics, various supplements, bio-electric baths, digestive enzymes, acupuncture, iridology, electro-dermal testing,

Oxytocin shots, vitamin B-12 shots, and much more. Little by little I have fought my way back to a functional level of health. With all that work, I have only managed to get up to a tolerable level. Many of the therapies only provide a short-term benefit, and then the therapy stops working. Because of that I continue alternative therapies.

That is where I was at when I decided to look into the Biotape™ treatments with you. Actually, I feel that I was led to you. I had heard about your pain treatments a year ago, but I didn't think that the treatments could help me because I don't have typical back pains or headaches. Recently, I experienced some health setbacks, so I began praying for guidance on what to do. One day, for no apparent reason, I decided to check out your web pages, even though I didn't think the therapy was something that could help me.

As I read your papers on the Chinese theory of pain, I began to realize that the four incisions in my midsection could be blocking the energy flow through my body and contributing to my health problems. I realized that even though the surgeries had accomplished their intended purpose, it was possible that my health problems were a side effect from those surgeries. That is when I decided to make an appointment with you.

I am so glad that I decided to call you. After you put the tape on my incisions, I immediately felt a difference. The burning pain in my arm diminished. The next day I felt great. Since putting the tape on, my sleep has improved, my energy is up, and the weird pains are barely there.

Thank you so much for your help and your work with Biotape™. The work you are doing and the knowledge you have is extremely important. I hope that you are sharing your knowledge with others. The world needs this knowledge. I have worked with numerous medical doctors and alternative therapists over the years. Most of them end up scratching their heads and telling me that I'm a mystery. I wasn't a mystery to you. You understood why I have had long-term health problems and you also offered a real solution. I am grateful for the benefits I have received from you and I am looking forward to continued improvement in my health.

Thank you,

Jim Johnson

P.S. I have been recommending you and your Biotape™ to everyone I know. My sister-in-law was experiencing severe pain in her arms from torn ligaments. I suggested she visit you. The next day she told me she had slept pain-free the whole night. It was a great relief for her.

Placing a single strip of Biotape™ along incisions is successful for treating post-surgical pain and even the pain known as reflex sympathetic dystrophy. I have had good success with women who have experienced health problems due to "tummy tuck" surgery. Taping incisions after breast enhancement or reduction surgery brings relief from the problems incident to those operations. A man who was paralyzed on his right side after hernia surgery and repair came to me in a wheelchair. The day after putting Biotape™ over his surgical incision, he "walked all over Salt Lake City."

I have also seen unusual success treating spider veins with Biotape™. I am indebted to Gary Kelson, who made the following discovery. He came to me after I had treated his wife for back pain to show me what he had done. When the tape came off his wife's back, Gary applied the tape to a large bruise that was actually a mass of spider veins on his leg. When he removed it, there was a strip through the middle of the bruise where the tape had been. The spider veins had totally disappeared. Other patients have obtained similar results.

Experience has shown that Biotape™, even when applied by an amateur over a scar or pain site, will give equal or better results than scar therapy or prolotherapy. Painful injections with a known carcinogen and/ or taking drugs are unnecessary. There is a better way to help even the most severely chronic, intractable pain.

Banana Peel *Will* Stop Headaches, Ann Landers
(the good doctor is wrong!)

A neurologist specializing in headache treatments responded to an Ann Landers column in which it was suggested that a banana peel across the forehead and the back of the neck would help relieve headaches, perhaps because of the potassium in the peel. The doctor stated, "Headache is not always a minor disorder that responds easily to such simple cures. Each month in the United States, approximately three million days are spent in bed by headache sufferers. Many of these people are in excruciating pain, unable to tolerate even the light from a bedside lamp or the sound of a child's step. Some vomit repeatedly. For them, trying to cure a headache with banana peels is like trying to irrigate the Sahara by spitting."

I have measured the electrical resistance at the pain site in more than eighteen thousand treatments, and can state categorically that pain is caused by the breaking, cutting, failure, or suppression of electrical signals between cells in living tissue. With headaches this often occurs across the forehead and back of the neck.

When I read the Ann Landers column, I couldn't run to the kitchen fast enough to get a banana. I wanted to find out how well banana peels conduct electrical signals. As I suspected after reading her article, banana peels are excellent conductors. Putting the inside of a banana peel next to the skin, one across the forehead and another across the back of the neck, may help to heal the root cause of many headaches by reconnecting the broken circuits causing the pain.

For the cost of a banana, you, my readers, can find out for yourself. The doctor's advice that banana peels cannot help headaches is wrong! Banana peels will stop many headaches (no matter how severe). You may look silly wearing a banana peel on your forehead, but it sure beats $400 botulism toxin injections or the cost of nerve suppressing medication.

My personal banana peel experience: "A very sharp knife up under my skull, just above my right eye." That's exactly how it felt to me in the middle of the night. I was on my way to Idaho, with a full schedule of patients to see the next day, but had stopped to see my ninety-year-old mother on the way. When I went to bed I had the hint of a headache. By the middle of the night, however, I woke up with the sharpest headache I have ever experienced. What could I do? I could see that I wasn't going to be sleeping that night. Then I remembered the bananas on the kitchen counter. I got one and laid the inside of the peel over my eyebrow and eyelid. Immediately, the second the peel touched my eyelid, the pain was gone! I could barely believe it. I took the peel off and as quickly as the pain had stopped, the sharp knife shot back up under my skull again.

It seemed impossible. How could it have happened that fast? I thought I was dreaming. For the sake of science and objectivity, I had to try it one more time. Removing the peel brought the same sharp knife and the same excruciating pain. Replacing the peel brought the same blessed, instant relief. I left the banana peel in place, went to sleep, woke up without a headache, and haven't had another headache in five years.

Whenever or wherever you hurt, try banana peels held in place with an Ace bandage. It will amaze you how much they help to relieve pain and correct its cause.

Banana Peels most assuredly can stop headaches, Ann Landers. I know that as well as I know the sun will come up in the morning.

Conductive Headache Bands

As a result, the Pain Research Institute has applied for a patent and is testing a number of conductive materials to produce a conductive "Headache Band." Only two of the first twenty chronic headache sufferers reported receiving no relief from the headbands. Following is a response from one of the patients:

> To Whom It May Concern,
>
> I have suffered severe headaches since 1967 when I fractured my back ejecting from a jet during combat in North Vietnam. I have the headaches almost twenty-four hours a day.
>
> About a month ago, Darrell gave me a headband to use for my headaches. These headbands are wonderful! I wear them almost constantly to prevent headaches—even while sleeping. I notice that while I am wearing it, I seldom have a headache. If I take it off, my headache is back within a minute.
>
> I have loaned my headband to a number of persons suffering from headaches. Sometimes within minutes they hand it back saying their headache is gone. I highly recommend these headbands to anyone suffering from headaches."
>
> Robert Houghton, Major USAF (Ret)

Subsequent to writing the above letter, Major Houghton injured his back and had severe pain (sciatica) clear to his foot. He taped his headband along the route of pain—from just below his knee to his foot. The pain disappeared. He also reported that after wearing the headbands for about three months, the headaches are now better and he doesn't have to wear the headband anymore. For the first time in twenty-six years, Robert Houghton is free of headaches!

Here is another Headache Band story:

August 13, 2002

Dear Darrell Stoddard,

I am writing to request another conductive headband. My mother, Susan T., purchased one from you a little over a year ago for my husband. He gets migraines three or four times a week and spends many hours in bed. Since he has been using the conductive headband he has spent next to zero hours down with a migraine. He often wears the headband all day long, but he is able to work, concentrate, and enjoy life more fully. I have witnessed the miracle of this headband almost daily.

I am now pregnant and seem to get headaches a little more often myself. The headband has made it possible for me to go on with life. Lately, my husband and I have taken turns wearing the headband. I have also lent the headband to friends who have had migraines or headaches. They have commented on the difference it makes the second they take it off.

As you can tell, our conductive headband has had TONS of use and is getting a little worn out. I have enclosed a check to purchase a new one. Thank you for the amazing change it has made in our lives.

Sincerely,

Sharina A.

Cedar City, Utah

To purchase a conductive Headache Band, see: *http:/ /www.healpain.net.*

Here are more tips for stopping headaches without drugs:

Dehydration is a major cause of headaches, because dehydration pulls water from the brain. This causes the electrical signals in the head to fail, which is the cause of pain. Drinking more water, with the chlorine removed by evaporation or through a carbon filter, could stop most of your headaches. (Distilled or reverse osmosis water may not work because too many of the minerals have been removed to conduct electrical signals.)

I was discussing the above phenomenon with Dr. Verl McBride, Ph.D., who has spent a lifetime successfully helping children and adults with learning disabilities by synchronizing the hemispheres of the brain using patterning exercises. Dr. McBride suggested another way to stop headaches: Put a patch over one eye. If it hasn't helped within several minutes, take it off and try the other eye. Placing a patch over one eye visually eliminates the disharmony of the brain's hemispheres that may be causing the headache. There are also exercises that do this. One is crawling on your hands and knees. Don't turn your head, but follow your hands with your eyes.

Another way to stop headaches is to place Biotape™ across the forehead. Biotape™ cannot be used over and over again like a conductive headband, but it is effective for the same reason: it reconnects broken electrical signals between cells in the forehead, the cause of headaches.

I treated an elderly woman with chronic migraine headaches using auricular therapy. Then I put a strip of Biotape™ across her forehead, telling her to try it for an hour or two. "Just see if it helps," I suggested. "You don't have to leave it on, because it will make you look strange." I saw her about ten days later. She still had the strip of black Biotape™ across her forehead. "You even wore it to church?" I asked. "Yes," she said. "I didn't care what anyone thought. That was the first time in years that I didn't have constant headaches."

"All truth goes through three stages: First, it is ridiculed.Then, it is violently opposed. Finally, it is accepted as self-evident."

—Schopenhauer

Notes

1. Swanson D. W., Swenson W. M., et al. *Mayo Clinic Proceedings* 51:401-408.

2. See complete study and references at: *http://www.garynull.com/ documents/dental/toxicanesthetics.htm.*

———

CHAPTER FOUR

It is Better to Wet Your Pants than to Live with Chronic Pain

Dehydration and/ or the lack of minerals is the number one cause of non-injury pain.

"Human progress has never been achieved with unanimous consent. Those who are enlightened first are compelled to pursue the light in spite of others."

—Christopher Columbus

ABSTRACT

It is Better to Wet Your Pants thank to Live with Chronic Pain. Confessions of a Soft Drink. Back Pain, Mountain Dew, and Biotape™. Preventing High Blood Pressure, Edema, Congestive Heart Failure, and Pain (what we should have learned from the cows sixty years ago). Fountain of Youth. Guidelines for the Kind of Water to Drink.

It is Better to Wet Your Pants than to Live with Chronic Pain

There was a time when I couldn't walk across the floor for a hundred dollars a step when I first got up in the morning. My injured left ankle hurt so bad that I would nearly pass out if I put weight on it. After hopping around on one foot for a while, I was finally able to hobble through the day. The thing that made my injury even more distressing was that I was a pain specialist who had stopped pain in more than nine thousand patients, but I couldn't help myself.

The regular morning runs I had been faithfully making for twenty-six years came to an end. The goal of running like Larry Lewis was now impossible. I had my foot X-rayed. There were no fractures or broken bones. I tried my own treatments, bioelectric and auricular therapy. It did nothing for the pain. I had orthotics made, had my ankle taped, did all of the exercises given to me by a podiatrist, shot my foot full of vitamins B-6 and B-12, and injected all of the trigger points with procaine. I took vitamins and minerals of all kinds, along with glucosamine sulfate, glucosamine hydrochloride, phenylalanine, blue-green algae, cod liver oil, flaxseed oil, nonfat yogurt, pygnoginal, shark cartilage, etc.

I knew better, but when all the natural stuff failed, I tried aspirin, Tylenol™, and a number of NSAIDs. Some of these made the pain more bearable, but as soon as I stopped taking them, it returned with a vengeance. I was obviously masking the pain and making myself vulnerable for further injury. For nine months I tried everything I could imagine short of narcotics, and by then I was becoming desperate.

Then, I read the book, *Your Body's Many Cries for Water,* by F. Batmanghelidj, M.D. I started drinking more water, or at least thought I was drinking more water, but my efforts weren't consistent enough to help me, and the pain continued.

Then one of my patients, an engineer, developed a water softener/ purification system that used potassium chloride instead of sodium chloride. He came to my house to test the water and do a demonstration. The demonstration included filling a bowl with water and showing how much chlorine it contained. He had me immerse my hand in the water and stir it for five minutes. Again the water was tested and the chlorine was gone. I was told that the chlorine had been absorbed into my hand as I stirred the water. This was why I needed a whole-house water conditioning system, not just something to purify my drinking water. Chlorine is toxic, and I was absorbing it even as I showered or bathed.

I later told Dr. Remington, with whom I work, about the demonstration, and he said, "Some of the chlorine may have been absorbed, but most of it evaporated. That is why they have to keep putting chlorine in a swimming pool— because it evaporates." He added, "If you want to solve that problem, let your drinking water sit overnight without a lid and all of the chlorine will evaporate."

I began to do this, and by the end of the day I could see by how much water remained, the amount of water I had not drunk. This routine reminded me to consistently drink more water, and lo and behold, the painful foot that had crippled me for nine months improved. Now I run every morning like I did before my injury. I learned as much about stopping pain through this experience as I have in a lifetime of study.

Batmanghelidj is right: When we are in pain, our body is "crying for water."

Besides the pain in my foot disappearing, another interesting change came into my life. Several times a day I found myself running to the bathroom like a child—something I haven't done for more than fifty years. One of these days I'm not going to make it, but it will be worth it. "It is better to wet your pants than to live with chronic pain." I should have known better. One of my father's favorite sayings was, "The extra water you drink when you take a pill does you more good than the pill."

Confessions of a Soft Drink

Not all fluids will provide us with the hydration we need. The following essay by Debbie Moody entitled "Confessions of a Soft Drink" (first published in 1986 in "Today's Herbs," a newsletter published by Woodland Books, Louise Tenney, editor) reveals the harmful effects of soft drinks. It was reprinted about ten years later in *Enrich* magazine. Since then, this is the only book with authorized permission to reprint the article. It reads as follows:

Hello. I am a humble, effervescent liquid. Humble? Well, that is debatable. Actually, I am quite proud of myself. Allow me to brag a little.

I fizz, sparkle, and bubble my way into thousands of people all over the world, every day. I HAVE MUCH POWER! I cause masses of humanity to make beelines for snack dispensers in plush, high-rise buildings. I stir men, women, and teenagers to dash into their cars late at night to speed to their nearest 24-hour convenience store.

To give me an appetizing brown tint, I contain caramel coloring, which has genetic effects and is a cancer causing suspect. I sometimes have polyethylene glycol as one of my ingredients. Glycol is used as antifreeze in automobiles, and as an oil solvent.

The bubbles and fizz with which I potently burn human insides is caused by my phosphoric acid. The phosphorus in the acid upsets the body's calcium-phosphorus ratio and dissolves calcium out of the bones. This can eventually result in OSTEOPOROSIS, a weakening of the skeletal structure, which can make one susceptible to broken bones. Also, the phosphorus fights with the hydrochloric acid in human stomachs and renders it ineffective. This promotes indigestion, bloating and gassiness in many individuals.

I offer a selection of three types of sweeteners, according to the customer's preference. The sweeteners are: Saccharin or Aspartame in the diet type, and sugar or corn syrup in my regular drinks. These substances enhance my appeal and come disguised as "good" for everyone. However, tastes can be deceiving! Let me explain.

SACCHARIN is an artificial sweetener, which has raised some concern about cancer in laboratory animals. There are warning labels on containers in which saccharin is an ingredient. ASPARTAME, the more common "diet" sweetener, has been linked to convulsions, depression, insomnia, irritability, weakness, dizziness, headaches, mood changes and mental retardation. SUGAR and CORN SYRUP can induce both

HYPOGLYCEMIA (low blood sugar), and HYPERG-
LYCEMIA (high blood sugar), in susceptible individuals. Hypoglycemia has been linked to mental illness
and hyperglycemia to diabetes. Sugar gives you a lift or
burst of energy, then sends you crashing down to severe
fatigue. To get another charge, more sugary drinks are
consumed. This pattern exhausts the adrenal glands
and leaves a person with a chronic tired feeling.

GORGEOUS! THAT'S WHAT I AM! I come
dressed in a shiny metal can in various colors and tints.
Sometimes I am silver, sometimes gold, sometimes
blue, red, etc. I beckon and dazzle shoppers as they
stroll past me in the supermarket. On a HOT DAY, I am
especially ATTRACTIVE, and hands reach for cases of
me to share with friends at picnics and parties. However, I am very tricky. My thirst quenching liquid,
which is alluringly encased in an aluminum can, contains traces of the same metal. The acid in the soft drink
eats away the aluminum, which floats around until it is
ingested by the consumer. Aluminum is a very toxic
substance and builds up in the human body. It has a
particular affinity for the brain and has been linked to
the degenerative senility affliction, ALZHEIMER'S
disease.

Many times humans think they can LOSE WEIGHT
by drinking me in the "diet" form. NOT SO! My high
sodium content helps them retain water in their bodies,
and they become edemic. The kidneys and bladder do
not function properly after a long habit of soft drink
intake. The sugar in me destroys the beneficial flora in
the colon and constipation results. This locks the
toxins in the body so they cannot be eliminated properly. The blood is not pure, as a result, and the cells are

affected. In order to lose weight, fat must be flushed from the cells. The enzymes responsible for aiding the process of fat release are paralyzed when they are poisoned, and so cannot do their job. People DEFEAT THEIR PURPOSE when they try to lose weight by drinking me.

In conclusion, I would like to admit there is not a smidgen of humility in me. I am very EGOTISTICAL! I am MASTER over much of the decision-making ability of the human race. HA! You don't believe me??? Look on school campuses, in city parks, at ball games, in business offices, at street corners...anywhere there are people... SEE YOU AROUND!

Back Pain, Mountain Dew, and Biotape™

Two men in their thirties came to me with severe, intractable low back pain. Both were scheduled for spinal surgery. Brandon, who was scheduled for a spinal fusion the following Friday, came to me on a Saturday evening. He had been unable to work for three years. Because of his bad back and because he could not provide for his family, his wife had divorced him.

I applied Biotape™ to Brandon's lower back in the same way I had done for thousands of patients. Then I added the standard auricular therapy for low back pain that I had done for seven years. Eighty-five percent of the pain was gone before Brandon left the room. By Sunday morning, one hundred percent of the pain was gone. On Monday morning, Brandon canceled his surgery. I saw Brandon three years later. He was managing a department at Home Depot. The good news was that he had remarried and was still pain-free. Brandon said his back occasionally bothered him a little and that he thought he would come back for another treatment, but it had never been bad enough to push him to follow through.

I did the exact same treatment on another man scheduled for back surgery, but neither the Biotape™ nor the auricular therapy helped. He got no relief. When I questioned this man, I found that he was drinking twelve to fourteen cans of Mountain Dew a day to keep himself going at his job as a construction worker. Caffeine (contained in the Mountain Dew) is a diuretic. People who drink it lose more fluid than they take in. You could drink gallons of a caffeinated drink a day and still be dehydrated.

Because Biotape™ may not help those who are dehydrated, I told the second man he would probably have to stop drinking Mountain Dew before I could help him. The man's surgery was postponed, and he returned about five weeks later with the news that he had finally "kicked the habit." "Now," he said, "see if you can stop my pain so I don't need surgery." This time the treatment worked, the surgery was postponed indefinitely, and he was able to continue his work.

If you suffer with chronic pain and consume caffeinated drinks, it is possible that you could become pain-free without drugs or treatment simply by "kicking the habit" and drinking more water.

Preventing High Blood Pressure, Edema, Congestive Heart Failure, and Pain
(what we should have learned from the cows sixty years ago)

Diuretics and salt-restricted diets are related to dehydration in the elderly. If patients are dehydrated due to taking diuretics, it is difficult to relieve their pain because electricity will not travel through dry tissue. Without salt or ionic minerals (calcium, magnesium, and potassium), water will not conduct a signal. To become pain-free, patients must drink enough water and minerals to connect the broken circuits that cause their pain.

"The cow's developed large ankles and were dying from water retention due to heart problems." These words were spoken by Phyllis Unice, who tells the following story:

When I was young I lived on a large ranch in Northern Utah. We all had a lot of chores to do every day. One of my chores was to watch and fill the salt and pepper shakers for the table. I remember that when I had to fill the saltshaker, I had to take a hammer to the cellar. I would use it to hit the cloth bag of salt to make it less lumpy, so I could get the salt out. Then the Morton Salt Company came out with a new kind of salt. The box had a picture of a little girl holding an umbrella on it, and under it, the caption, "When it Rains, it Pours." This indicated that the salt was different, that it would not lump or cake.

My father and the other ranchers in the area put out large blocks of salt in the corrals and pastures for the cattle to lick. We called them "salt licks." Soon after the new salt was developed, my father's cows and the cows of other ranchers began to die. The cows developed large ankles and were dying from water retention due to heart problems. This was of great concern to the ranchers. The ranchers asked the animal science professors at Utah State University to investigate. Finally, what the investigation found was that the only thing that had changed in the cattle's diet was the salt. The Morton Salt Company produced all of the saltlicks, and the company had switched to saltlicks made from white salt that had been heated in a kiln. No one had noticed that there was a difference in the salt, as the salt licks looked the same, although perhaps whiter in color.

Needless to say, the ranchers changed back to the natural pink saltlicks, salt that hasn't been kiln-heated. When we changed back, the animals improved and we had no more problems. However, the salt you buy in the grocery store, for yourself, is still heated in a kiln and has aluminum anti-caking agents added to keep it from sticking together and to make it pure white. Salt in its natural state is important for good health because it helps regulate the way the body maintains moisture levels in the cells. The heating and the aluminum anti-caking agents change the salt to a product that is not good and produces in people the same symptoms that occurred in the animals.

If the cows had been people, then or now, we would have put them on a salt-restricted diet and given them a diuretic. Putting the cows on a salt-restricted diet and giving them a diuretic would have killed them.

Natural salt (salt that does *not* pour when it rains) absorbs moisture. The absorption of moisture is what makes it cake. This is purely theoretical, but I believe *natural* salt in the body pulls healthy moisture *into* the cells, helping to maintain the sodium-potassium balance vital to all cellular function. Table salt (that *does* pour when it rains) does not absorb moisture. Too much unnatural salt may cause the body to retain unhealthy moisture in the extra-cellular spaces. We call this edema. The wrong kind of salt could also cause dehydration, because not enough fluid is pulled into the cells.

I believe it is possible for cells to be simultaneously dehydrated and have edema (too much fluid outside the cells). Doctors tend to overlook this possibility when they treat hypertension (high blood pressure) and congestive heart failure by prescribing diuretics. The diuretic may reduce the blood pressure and eliminate edema, but it also upsets the delicate sodium-potassium balance in the cells.

As far as I know, all of the studies that have shown how excessive salt intake can lead to high blood pressure, water retention (edema), congestive heart failure, and a host of other diseases, have been done with the *wrong* kind of salt. The very fact that outside of the body one kind of salt cakes (absorbs moisture) and the other doesn't should tell us to expect that the effects of the two different types of salt to be different.

What a wonderful opportunity for new research. Could natural salt contribute to good health by hydrating the cells and preventing edema? Could too much unnatural salt cause high blood pressure, edema, congestive heart failure, and pain? I have found that edematous tissue is a poor conductor of electricity, and suppressed or broken electrical circuits are the cause of pain. We should have learned a lesson from the cows sixty years ago. It may be the *kind* of salt we eat that causes serious, even fatal, disease, not how much salt we consume.

Fountain of Youth

Ponce de Leon, who accompanied Columbus on his second voyage in 1500, learned of a fountain with magical ingredients that could restore youth. Searching for the mystical fountain, he discovered and named Florida on Easter. The fountain he was looking for was not an herb or vegetable or exotic fruit. It was a fountain. He had that part right. Five hundred years later, I believe the fountain of youth is pure water, which contains the ionic minerals calcium, sodium, magnesium, and potassium.

For evidence that water is the fountain of youth, consider what happens when people don't get enough. I believe dehydration (and/ or lack of minerals) is the final cause of death for most old people. An elderly person weighing 150 pounds has about seven liters less water than a young person of the same weight. As a result of this lower water content, elderly individuals can become dehydrated more quickly. Dehydration is one of the reversible causes of dementia.[1]

Older people reduce their water intake because they think it makes them go to the bathroom too often. (The reason they have the urge to urinate is not because of a full bladder but because their urine is too concentrated.) When they drink less water, their urine becomes even more concentrated, and they find they have the urge to go even more often. If old people would drink more water, they would have the urge to go to the bathroom less often, because they would then feel the need to urinate only when the bladder was full. Knowing this and acting upon it will save more lives than any other single action.

It is an accepted and indisputable fact that we are "brain dead" when there is no more electricity crossing the brain. Heart failure comes when there is no more electricity in the heart muscles to make the heart pump. Every other function, organ, and cell in the body dies without the minute electrical signals that are the living part of every cell. We must have water *and* minerals, or the electrical signals fail and cells die.

Guidelines For the Kind of Water to Drink

Do not drink distilled water. Distilled water is electrically dead. The distillation process removes all the minerals. Without minerals, water will not conduct the electrical signals requisite to the life of *every* cell and the pain-free functioning of the human body. Drinking distilled water may be one of the worst things you can do for your health. (See: "Early Death Comes from Drinking Distilled Water" at: *http://www.mercola.com/.*) Reverse osmosis water is only slightly better than distilled water because again, many minerals are removed in the processing.

The last time I was at the National Institute of Health, I was shown a chart that plotted the incidence of heart disease and water, hard or soft. Where the water is softer, there is more heart disease. Where the water is harder, there is less heart disease. Hard water contains more minerals; soft water has fewer minerals. Distilled water has *no* minerals. We must consume minerals if the heart, brain, and all other organs and cells are to function properly.

Do not drink chlorinated water without allowing the chlorine to evaporate first. Chlorine is a toxin. It's put in water to kill germs. It kills houseplants and goldfish too. It's not good for you either. To dechlorinate your water, let it sit out uncovered for two hours. Most of the chlorine will evaporate in that time.

What about bottled water? We have tested most brands of bottled drinking water available locally, and believe that in most cities, simply allowing the chlorine to evaporate from water used for cooking, drinking, and bathing will provide you with water that is as good to drink as ninety-five percent of the bottled water you buy.

Next best, however, is to drink water that has gone through an activated carbon filter, if the filter is changed as often as prescribed. These filters remove chlorine and most other impurities without removing the minerals. Ideally, the filter should be equipped with something that tells you when it needs to be changed.

If you are coping with pain, the next best thing you could do after filtering your water is to add ionic minerals to it. The Pain Research Institute has formulated a Fountain of Youth Hydration/ Arthritis Formula containing the following ingredients: vitamin C (as ascorbic acid), magnesium and potassium aspartate, cetyl myristoleate, MSM, glucosamine sulfate, and bromelain. Because these minerals are dissolved in the water, they will be much easier to absorb than when they are in pill form. Many pills never dissolve, especially in the elderly, who suffer from malabsorption. People who pump out septic tanks will tell you they are often full of undissolved pills. In hospitals they are called bedpan bullets because they go right through elderly patients. You cannot be pain-free if you are dehydrated or if you don't get enough ionic minerals.

> *"The jury is composed of the old guard who, as history teaches us, have a vested interest in protecting the status quo, no matter what the cost in human lives."*
> —Robert Barefoot

Our Biotape™ Hydration Formula is available from: Smart Inventions, Inc., 6319 E. Alondra Blvd., Paramount, CA 90723-3750; call toll free 1-800-977-6336.

Notes

1. *Dehydration in the Elderly,* University of Iowa *Family Practice Handbook,* Fourth Edition, Chapter 9, available at: *http://millennium.fortunecity.com/firemansam/328/cu198dehydration.htm.*

CHAPTER FIVE

More Preventable Causes of Pain

Fibromyalgia, Chronic Fatigue Syndrome, and Alzheimer's Disease

"Paradoxical as it may seem, God means not only to make us good, but to make us also happy, by sickness, disaster, and disappointment."

—C. A. Bartol

ABSTRACT

Synopsis. What are Fibromyalgia and Chronic Fatigue Syndrome? What is Alzheimer's Disease? Possible Cause—the Aluminum Factor. Diet and Prevention—Confirming Scientific Research. Why are Fibromyalgia and Chronic Fatigue Syndrome New? Summary.

101

Synopsis

The painful disease known as fibromyalgia is now epidemic and we know that few diseases are as emotionally painful for the patient or his or her loved ones than Alzheimer's disease. The following words from a medical journal I was reading leapt off the page: "Chronic fatigue syndrome might represent early or evolving Alzheimer's disease." Is chronic fatigue syndrome (and fibromyalgia that nearly always goes with it) emerging Alzheimer's disease in young people? Could there be a connection between fibromyalgia (FM)/ chronic fatigue syndrome (CFS) and Alzheimer's disease (AD)? After reviewing more than a hundred articles on the subject, what follows is one of few *attempts* to explain the cause of these new and mystifying diseases together with new insights into the cause of Alzheimer's. Most articles say the cause of FM/ CFS is unknown, and many say the diseases are incurable. I believe both statements are false.

What are Fibromyalgia and Chronic Fatigue Syndrome?

Fibromyalgia and chronic fatigue syndrome (also known as chronic fatigue immune deficiency syndrome [CFIDS]) seem to be new diseases. It appears that neither of them existed fifty years ago. Or, if they did exist, they were not identified or named. Now these diseases are epidemic. According to the American College of Rheumatology, fibromyalgia affects three to six million Americans. Seven times as many women are afflicted with CFS than men.

Many doctors debate whether these diseases do exist, because there are no widely recognized medical tests to identify either of them. They are identified simply by their symptoms. Some claim that we have created FM/ CFS by naming them. It is reassuring for patients to put a name on their symptoms even if we don't know the cause or what to do about them.

In the medical clinic where I have worked for thirteen years we have seen more than one thousand patients with symptoms of FM/ CFS. When admitted to the clinic, every patient fills out a symptom checklist describing 169 symptoms. It addition to the "hurt all over" and "tired all the time" symptoms, almost all FM/ CFS patients also check, "difficulty concentrating," "trouble thinking clearly," "indecisiveness," "confusion," "memory disturbances," and "learning disabilities." If this isn't "early or evolving Alzheimer's disease," many of the symptoms are still the same. The causes may also be related.

What is Alzheimer's Disease?

"Alzheimer's disease is *a degenerative disease of the brain from which there is no recovery.* Slowly and inexorably, the disease attacks nerve cells in all parts of the cortex of the brain . . . About half of the people in nursing homes and almost half of all people over eighty-five have Alzheimer's disease. It is now *the fourth leading cause of death in adults.* Almost two million Americans have Alzheimer's, and unless effective methods for prevention and treatment are developed, it will reach epidemic proportions by the middle of the next century, afflicting over eight million people." (emphasis added)[1] This chapter will show that the possibility of recovery from Alzheimer's disease is not as bleak as the above definition. Knowing the cause of FM/ CFS and AD offers hope of prevention *and* treatment.

Possible Cause: The Aluminum Factor

In the 1980s, aluminum was suspected to be one of the causes of Alzheimer's disease when aluminum of higher than normal amounts was found by autopsy in the brains of people who had died from the disease. To test the theory, animals were given aluminum in different forms. The experimental injection of aluminum into animals did cause neurofibrillary tangles in the brain, but they were different from the neurofibrillary tangles seen in the brains of AD patients. Therefore the theory was discounted and abandoned. Although it is widely recognized that aluminum is a neurological toxin, most experts today either believe the excessive aluminum in the brains of AD patients is the *effect* of the disease and not the *cause,* or they believe the aluminum was not measured properly. In *Scientific American,* an Alzheimer specialist answering the question, "Is Alzheimer's disease related to aluminum exposure?" called such a notion a "myth." In explaining how the myth got started, the doctor ironically still presented evidence linking aluminum to AD. [2]

Other scientists have published new research in peer review scientific journals that still promotes aluminum as one of the causes of Alzheimer's. The challenge is to discover or prove what makes the aluminum deposit in the brain. Theories have been proposed and compelling evidence offered to explain the mechanism of why and how aluminum does so.

Diet and Prevention: Confirming Scientific Research

Aluminum is the third most common element on the earth's crust; thus small amounts of aluminum may be present in the water we drink and in the food we eat. It is impossible to eliminate all aluminum from the diet. Because of this, people have always developed Alzheimer's, whereas FM/ CFS seem to be new diseases. In AD, the amount of aluminum consumed seems to make no difference. Even people with very low levels of aluminum consumption get Alzheimer's. However, there are studies to indicate that the incidence of AD increases with the amount of aluminum in the water supply. Alum (potassium aluminum sulfate) is added to most culinary drinking water systems as a clearing agent.[3] The World Health Organization recommends that the amount of aluminum present in drinking water remain below two hundred micrograms per liter.

A 1996 study by D. R. C. McLachlan et al found a correlation between the level of aluminum present in drinking water and the number of diagnosed Alzheimer's cases. This study concluded that between 15,180 and 26,910 of the estimated 66,000-117,000 cases of AD might have been prevented if aluminum concentration in the municipal water supply had been kept below one hundred micrograms per liter.[4]

A year 2000 study from France that followed 2,700 individuals for an eight-year period showed that a concentration of aluminum in drinking water above 0.1 milligrams per liter may be a risk factor for contracting dementia and Alzheimer's.[5]

It has also been found that cola drinks in aluminum cans contain sixteen times as much aluminum as the aluminum concentration in local tap water. Non-cola soft drinks in aluminum cans contained twenty-three times as much aluminum. The leaching of aluminum into soft drinks increased with the level of the soft drink's acidity. Beer is also highly acidic and is now available in aluminum cans. In the past, beer came only in glass bottles.[6]

The island of Guam has much aluminum in its soil and consequently much aluminum in its drinking water. When a disease similar to Alzheimer's dementia was prevalent even in the young people, the government suspected aluminum. The water was purified and the young people are no longer afflicted. It has been accepted in Guam that aluminum in the drinking water causes dementia.[7]

William B. Grant, Ph.D. has written several articles addressing the aluminum/ AD theory. In one such paper he presents a compelling theory of what makes aluminum deposit in the brains of people with AD.[8] In another he states, "Aluminum is strongly bound to oxygen unless it is dissolved in a strong acid.... Aluminum oxide is basically inert, so when ingested will pass through the digestive system intact unless the digestive system is acidic from over-consumption of acid-forming foods such as fats and proteins, with possibly some contribution from highly processed carbohydrates."[9]

According to Dr. Grant, "Increasing the consumption of calcium supplements when eating acid-forming foods might reduce the absorption of aluminum. A better solution may be to include fewer acid-forming and more alkaline-forming foods in the diet."[10]

Dr. Grant also indicated that other metals and elements aside from aluminum were found in higher than normal concentrations in the brains of autopsied Alzheimer's patients. These metals include silver, cobalt, iron, mercury, scandium, and sodium, with mercury being the highest of all. The alkali metals, cesium, potassium, and rubidium were found to be lower than normal.

Dr. Grant's summary reads as follows:

> There is strong evidence that the incidence and prevalence of AD is affected by diet, with high risk factors found to include alcohol, fat, refined carbohydrates, salt, and total caloric consumption, and preventative factors found to include antioxidants, essential trace minerals, estrogen for postmenopausal women, fish and fish oil, and antiinflammatory therapeutic agents.... Thus, healthy diets should be considered the first line of defense against both the development and progression of AD, as well as all other chronic degenerative diseases. The finding that the highest correlation between diet and AD incidence and prevalence is

found 3-5 years before the study period suggests that diet modifications late in life can still affect the risk of developing AD.

George M. Tamari, Ph.D., lists twenty-three diseases linked to aluminum toxicity, including Alzheimer's, pain, weakness, fatigue, and aching muscles. (Sounds like a description of FM/ CFS.) Tamari reports that people whose diets are "deficient in calcium and/ or zinc will absorb more aluminum than well fed subjects" and that "antagonistic elements, like zinc and calcium, will replace aluminum." In conclusion he states, "By ingesting food rich in the deficient element, or by using food supplements, the unwanted toxic elements may be 'replaced' by antagonistic nutritional elements." A zinc deficiency may cause aluminum to deposit in the brain, but excessive amounts of zinc may promote formation of amyloid plaques in the brain, a characteristic of AD. Too little or too much zinc could contribute to AD. Fluoride is also an antagonistic element of aluminum, but is not recommended because of its toxicity.[11]

A 1993 study by Domingo et al reveals something interesting. Eight groups of mice were given eight different acids commonly found in the human diet in their drinking water for one month. The mice were all killed, and the amount of aluminum measured in their bones and four of their major organs. The acids actually *caused* aluminum (from the water and food they had consumed) to *deposit* in the bones and organs of the body, including the brain, instead of chelating the aluminum out! The study concludes, "Because of the wide presence and consumption of the above dietary constituents, in order to prevent aluminum accumulation and toxicity, we suggest a drastic limitation of human exposure to aluminum."[12]

Malic acid, all of the acids used in the above study, amino acids from meat, fats, and protein—all of these may cause aluminum that would otherwise pass through the body to deposit in the bone, organs, and *brain*. Alkaline drinking water, essential minerals (including calcium, magnesium, and potassium), and alkaline-forming foods may prevent this from happening.

It has also been discovered that low doses of fluoride (the equivalent of 1.0 ppm, the "optimal" dose added to drinking water to prevent dental cavities) may cause aluminum to deposit in the brain. *Brain Research,* a peer review medical journal, reported in 1998 that the amount of aluminum deposited in the brain of low-dose fluoride-treated rats was *double* that of the controls! (Fluoride, which is antagonistic to aluminum, made the aluminum bio-available to cross the blood-brain barrier.)[13] Visit any Alzheimer's ward or elderly care facility and ask yourself, "Do we really need fluoride in our drinking water?"

A new study led by North Carolina State University offers great promise for *treatment*. Researchers found that aluminum levels in the brains of laboratory mice decreased by eighty percent after the mice were given supplemental doses of a protein called peptide YY. The sharp drop in aluminum levels occurred after injecting the mice with the protein supplements for just three days.[14]

There is enough new and old evidence in scientific journals to link aluminum to AD. Therefore we should *reconsider* aluminum as one of the possible causes of Alzheimer's disease. That the neurofibrillary tangles induced in animals were not the same as the neurofibril-lary tangles seen in the brains of AD patients, or that people with low aluminum intake still get AD, or that the aluminum in the brain was not measured properly, is not justification to abandon the theory.

Why are Fibromyalgia and Chronic Fatigue Syndrome New?

The fact that FM/ CFS are new diseases indicates that our intake of aluminum must have increased in the last fifty years. The two new and worst offenders are soft drinks and beer in aluminum cans and antiperspirants in most deodorants.

In the olden days, fifty years ago or so, soft drinks were not sold in aluminum cans. Rather, they were available only in returnable, refillable glass bottles. In addition, other than a few people who were addicted to drinking Coca Cola, people did not drink soft drinks on a daily basis. The apparent addiction to soft drinks we see today in almost all teenagers and young people did not exist. These young people are our FM/ CFS generation.

To understand my theory of how aluminum from antiperspirants may be one of the causes of both AD and FM/ CFS, one needs to learn about the skin's function. We usually think of the skin as something that holds us together, but the skin is a complex organ that performs an astounding number of functions. It is the largest organ in the body. A single square inch of skin contains approximately nineteen million cells, including 650 sweat glands, one hundred sebum or oil glands, sixty-five hair follicles, nineteen thousand sensory cells, and as much as thirteen feet of microscopic blood vessels. The skin helps regulate blood pressure, protects us from heat and cold, and protects the body from the invasion of harmful bacteria. The skin absorbs oxygen and emits carbon dioxide, and it manufactures vitamin D and a myriad of complex chemicals to protect and keep us well.

The skin is also an organ of elimination through perspiration/ respiration. The four organs of elimination are the bowels, kidneys, lungs, and skin. The function of perspiration is not only to cool the body but to eliminate toxins from the body. This is mostly done from under the arms. The smell is evidence of that fact. When the elimination of even the small amounts of toxins are stopped by the absorption of aluminum in antiperspirants (along with aluminum from other sources), the result, I believe, is fibromyalgia and chronic fatigue syndrome. Any other mineral, chemical, or stone from the health food store that claims to stop perspiration would also be harmful. It is okay to use a deodorant, but if it says *"antiperspirant,"* it should be discarded.

If we understand the skin's elimination function, the very word "antiperspirant" should give us concern. Would we take into our body or use anything called "anti-bowel movement" to prevent elimination because our feces smells bad? Would we take or use anything called "anti-urination" to keep us from voiding because the smell of urine is unpleasant? Last of all, would we take or use anything called "anti-breathing" to prevent bad breath? Using an antiperspirant makes as much sense! Remember, deodorant is not the suspected culprit. It is the antiperspirant (aluminum) added to almost all deodorants that is the problem. If perspiration gives you a bad odor, you should get down on your knees and thank God that your skin has eliminated whatever caused the smell.

I believe if you were to cover your body in antiperspirant, thereby stopping the cycle of respiration and perspiration, you would become ill in a short time. You wouldn't need to wait for FM/ CFS or AD to develop. In the James Bond movie *Goldfinger,* an actor was painted in a gold substance. The substance could only be left on for a short time, because blocking the respiration/ perspiration functions of the skin was too deadly. The actor could have suffocated to death, since the skin would have been unable to take in oxygen and give off carbon dioxide, which it does much like the lungs do.

It's true that the amount of toxins eliminated by the skin is very small compared to the amount of toxins eliminated by other organs. Still, I don't think the importance of the skin's elimination/ respiration functions has been adequately investigated. Just as the kidneys cannot do the job of the bowels or the lungs, the other organs of elimination cannot replace or do what the skin does.

Fifty years ago, before the discovery that aluminum stops perspiration, women wore plastic shields and/ or pads under their arms to protect their clothing, and used powder or cornstarch to absorb sweat. They also wore fragrance to mask odor. People did not have antiperspirants in those days, and neither did we seem to have unrelenting fatigue or so much nonarthritic pain as to render them completely non-functional.

Before antiperspirants, my father, a smoker, had big white circular stains made by perspiration under the arms of all his shirts. The cloth in those circles would rot, ruining the shirts. Perspiration is how my father eliminated the nicotine and other harmful substances he took into his body when he smoked. You could smell the cigarettes when my mother washed his shirts. I think the smell was not only from the smoke getting into his clothes but from the toxins eliminated in the perspiration under his arms. The average life expectancy of a male smoker is currently seventy-two years. If my father had used antiperspirants, the cigarette toxins would *not* have been eliminated. I don't believe he would have lived to the age of seventy-nine.

Do people who do not use antiperspirants get FM/CFS symptoms? Yes. The same symptoms can be caused by dehydration and/ or a lack of essential minerals. Of course, these things are much easier to correct. In most patients the symptoms described are a combination of the two. Do all people who use antiperspirants get FM/ CFS? No. Contracting these diseases depends on how effectively a person's body can eliminate aluminum.

People in the health food industry have been telling us for fifty years not to use aluminum cookware, baking powder that contains aluminum, and more recently, antacids containing aluminum. They have also decried consumption of soft drinks sold in aluminum cans. I believe the amount of aluminum that goes into the tissues from such sources is minimal compared to the doses most people rub under their arms every morning—a dose that is absorbed directly into the muscles, ligaments, and tendons, the same fibrous body tissues where fibromyalgia manifests. You may absorb and retain as much aluminum from one application of antiperspirant as you would from using aluminum cookware over a lifetime.

There is no experimental evidence to prove that aluminum in antiperspirants causes FM/ CFS. I am simply presenting a hypothesis worth considering. We don't need to guess how the deodorant companies, soft drink manufacturers, and fluoride proponents will respond. Those with FM/ CFS can try the suggestions below and find out for themselves. The remedies I have suggest cost nothing. I have nothing to sell. Experience has shown that avoiding aluminum may help FM/ CFS within weeks.

Summary

I now conclude with the same question with which I began: "Are fibromyalgia and chronic fatigue syndrome Alzheimer's disease in young people? Is there a connection between FM/ CFS and AD?" If I am correct about aluminum being one of the causes of both diseases, the consequences are staggering. There could be an epidemic of Alzheimer's like the world has never known, as the generation using antiperspirants, drinking soft drinks, and consuming fluoride in their drinking water and toothpaste ages. It not only foreshadows terrible things to come, but conversely offers hope of preventing one of the most tragic of all diseases, AD, and sparing others from the disabling effects of FM/ CFS.

If I am wrong, there are still plenty of reasons to avoid aluminum. As far as I know, no one has ever presented evidence that aluminum in *any* amount is good for the health of trees, plants, animals, or humans. Most just say that aluminum in small amounts does no harm. No one even argues that aluminum in any amount is beneficial. Innumerable articles and studies claim that aluminum is harmful to the body.

If you believe that aluminum could be one of the causes of FM/ CFS or don't want to take a chance, the message for you to take home is this: you may be able to prevent and/ or reverse the effects of fibromyalgia, chronic fatigue syndrome, Alzheimer's disease, and other degenerative diseases by doing the following:

1. Don't use antiperspirants.
2. Don't drink soft drinks from aluminum cans.
3. Don't use antacids that contain aluminum.
4. Don't use baking powder containing aluminum.
5. Don't drink your tap water unless the chlorine has been removed.
6. Don't drink fluoridated water or use fluoride toothpaste.
7. Don't use *buffered* aspirin or other medications if they contain aluminum.
8. Don't use malic acid to treat FM/ CFS because this may cause aluminum to deposit in the brain.

Note: This chapter is a condensed version of the article, "Fibromyalgia, Chronic Fatigue, Alzheimer's: Causes and Treatments." To view the entire article, see *http://www.healpain.net.*

"Yesterday is but today's memory, and tomorrow is today's dream."

— Kahlil Gibran

Notes

1. "What is Alzheimer's Disease?" For the full article see: *http://my.webmd.com/content/article/1680.50324.*

2. *Scientific American* at: *http://www.sciam.com/askexpert/medicine/medicine22.html.*

3. Re: the alum added to drinking water issue, see: *http://www.awwa.org/govtaff/aluminpa.htm.*

4. McLachlan D.R, et al. "Risk for Neuropathologically Confirmed Alzheimer's Disease and Residual Aluminum in Municipal Drinking Water Employing Weighted Residential Histories." *Neurology.* 46 (1996): 401-405.

5. "Aluminum in Drinking Water": *American Journal of Epidemiology* 2000; 152:59-66.

6. Dragen J. M., Dickeson J. E., Tynan, P. F. et al. "Aluminum Beverage Cans as a Dietary Source of Aluminum," *Med J Aust* 1992; 156: 604-5.

7. Batmanghelidj F. *Your Body's Many Cries for Water,* pp.37-8.

8. Grant, W. B., "Alzheimer's, Acid Rain, and Aluminum," at: *http://www.healpain.net/.*

9. Grant, W. B., "Aluminum Accumulates in Body with High Acid Diet," *Townsend Letter for Doctors,* June 1999, p.92.

10. Grant, W. B., "Dietary Links to Alzheimer's Disease" at: *http://www.mc.uky.edu/adreview/Vol2/Grant/Grant.htm - top.*

11. Tamari, George M., "Aluminum—Toxicity and Prevention," *Townsend Letter for Doctors & Patients,* Feb/ Mar 1999, pp. 98-100.

12. Domingo, J. L., Gomez, M., Sanchez, D. J., Llobet, J. M., Corbella, J, "Effect of Various Dietary Constituents on Gastrointestinal Absorption of Aluminum from Drinking Water and Diet," *Res Commun Chem Pathol Pharmacol,* 1993 Mar, 79:3, pp. 377-80.

13. Verner, J. A., et al. "Chronic Administration of Aluminum Flouride to Rats in Drinking Water: Alterations in Neuronal and Cerebrovascular Integrity," *Brain Research*, Vol. 784:1998.

14. "Peptide YY for Chelating AL from the Brain," *http://www.mercola.com/2000/aug/6/peptide_aluminum.htm*

CHAPTER SIX

—•—

Conclusion

*"If all the drugs were thrown into the ocean,
it would be all the worse for the fishes and all
the better for mankind."*
—Oliver Wendell Holmes

The above statement attributed to Oliver Wendell Holmes is only partly true. In my estimation, if even *half* of all drugs were thrown into the ocean, it would be all the worse for the fishes and all the better for mankind.

The above statement brings me to what I believe is a major flaw in the thinking of most human beings, including doctors, health care providers, and patients. Some people (alternative medicine devotees) believe all drugs are harmful; they would die before taking them. Others believe orthodox medicine can do no wrong and that medical doctors do not make mistakes. Such patients have implicit faith in their doctors, who believe that unless they have read it in the *New England Journal of Medicine* or the *Journal of the American Medical Association*, it is pure quackery. People either think the letters M.D. stand for "Minor Deity" or "More Dangerous." *Both* positions are wrong, but nearly everyone falls firmly on one side or the other.

Because I have been critical of many orthodox medical practices in this book, I would like to point out how wrong it is to think that alternative medicine (herbs and vitamins and *no* drugs—the health food route) is the *only* way to go, and that all MDs and orthodox medications are bad.

One of my patients had a brother-in-law who was the vice-president of a bank. His wife was convinced that she could cure her husband's ulcers with cayenne pepper. The cayenne did not cure the ulcers, and the man bled to death internally. Orthodox medicine would most certainly have saved his life. With the discovery of the helicobacter pylori bacteria as a major cause of ulcers, orthodox medicine, knowing how to treat ulcers, has almost eliminated that scourge from the face of the earth, just as it eliminated smallpox and polio before it. I do not believe that the cayenne caused or worsened the man's bleeding ulcers. But the cayenne cure did keep the man from getting the treatment that would have saved his life. Modern orthodox medicine has eliminated the smallpox epidemics that killed millions of people. We no longer see hospital wards filled with iron lungs. In modern industrialized nations, the tuberculosis sanitariums have disappeared. Flu epidemics no longer kill endless numbers of people. There are no more cholera or typhoid epidemics in the industrialized world. Pneumonia is no longer the death sentence it once was. Penicillin and other antibiotics (although overused) have probably saved many of our lives at one time or another. Let's not throw the baby out with the bathwater or cast out our medical saviors in favor of the herbs sold in health food stores that are themselves drugs. Marijuana, opium, cocaine, and heroin are, after all, herbs. You could even call them "natural." Just because something is natural does not necessarily make it better than a chemical medication. Don't let anyone tell you that herbs are natural and that no one has ever been harmed by taking them. Innumerable numbers of people die every year from using the herbs I listed above.

The publication of a study in the July 2000 *Journal of the American Medical Association* was a difficult pill for the orthodox medical folks to swallow. This study claimed that *doctors* cause 225,000 deaths per year in the U.S. That makes doctors the third leading cause of death in the U.S. each year, just after cancer and heart disease, and far ahead of the next leading cause, cerebrovascular disease (stroke).

The next pill may be even more difficult to swallow: If you acknowledge John Gofman's monumental study on the number of cancer and heart disease deaths caused by an accumulated exposure to medical X-rays, doctors become the number one cause of death in the U.S. Gofman, one of the premier scientists of all time (whose medical and scientific credentials fill five pages), estimates that 250,000 lives could be saved each year in the United States if medical X-ray exposure was reduced by fifty percent. Gofman shows how this can easily be done with NO loss of vital information (See: *Cancer Alert—A Major Cause of Cancer and Heart Disease Your Doctor, Dentist, or Chi ropractor Does Not Want You To Know,* and *Better than a Cure for Breast Cancer* at *http://www.healpain.net.*)

If these statistics are to improve, changes must be made in our health care system. As Joseph Mercola, one of the best and most outspoken medical doctors in the U.S. has said, "The medical paradigm is broken and must be fixed." This requires change. Niels Bohr used even stronger words to reveal how scientific knowledge progresses: "Science advances funeral by funeral."

The purpose of this book is to help you become pain-free for life and to change the way Western medicine defines and treats pain. For either of these goals to be realized requires the recognition that the traditional approach to pain may not only be harmful but profoundly wrong. It will take a paradigm shift to go from treating the pain signal to treating the cause of pain. We have offered innumerable clinical treatments and anecdotal evidence to validate the Chinese definition of pain and disease. We have also presented a method to scientifically confirm with randomized, double-blind, placebo-controlled studies the Chinese definition of pain.

One last story to illustrate the desperate need to change the way Western medicine defines and treats pain: Ten years ago, eighty-one-year-old Melpha Squires came tottering into my office with her walker. A neurologist had told her family that she would have to use the walker for the rest of her life. After my treatment to connect the broken circuits that caused her pain, she walked out of the room without any aid, and the next day walked all over town without her walker. Seven months later, she walked briskly into the room to see me for pain that had returned. She still didn't need her walker or cane. Each treatment brought pain relief that lasted about six months. When a treatment given in 1994 did not help, she had hip replacement surgery. After the hip replacement, she was able to walk without a walker or cane for eight years, because she was not taking pain medication. This morning (December 4, 2002) she told me that her artificial hip has worn out and that she needs another hip replacement. She recently began to use a cane. Now ninety-one years old, Mrs. Squires still does not need a walker.

Our rest homes, retirement, and assisted-living centers are full of elderly people who are barely able to walk. Rather, they totter with the aid of their walkers. Much of their disability is caused by pain medication and sedatives. You cannot suppress the pain signal, the sensory nerves, the central nervous system, or dehydrate the body without suppressing motor nerves and causing loss of function. Pain medication, sedatives, and diuretics cause some of the dementia we see in the elderly. Pain medication, sedatives, and diuretics cause much of the constipation in the aged. Nearly all of the gastrointestinal bleeding in the elderly is caused by pain medication. Loss of liver function, kidney function, and even lung and heart function may be caused by pain medication and sedatives. There is a better way to treat and even heal pain than using pain medication and sedatives.

My wife and I do volunteer work at an assisted living center full of elderly people barely able to walk. Most of the residents take countless pain medications every day. I have recently returned from China. I was struck (as I am every time I go to China) by the contrast in the state of our elderly. At daybreak, every park in China is full of elderly people doing beautiful, graceful Tai Chi exercises. They are not tottering through the park with walkers or being wheeled in wheelchairs. Could it be that they know something we don't?

Pain is the blockage of Chi, the cutting, breaking, suppression, or failure of electrical connections between cells. Pain is healed when the broken connections are reestablished. You now have the knowledge of what pain is and how to heal your pain, the pain of loved ones, or the pain of patients.

Our impossible dream will come true when Western medicine changes the way pain is defined and treated. This will happen only when many randomized, double-blind, placebo-controlled studies by independent researchers demonstrate what I have outlined in this book. Through an understanding of what pain is will come the knowledge to heal pain, not just to suppress the pain signal.

Whether you are a health care provider or a victim of pain, it is now up to you.

Joy will
Follow pain
And the amount of joy
Depends on how much and
How long you have been afflicted.

Exquisite joy will follow suffering
And the height and breadth and depth
Of that joy is determined by how long
And how much you have suffered.

Justice demands that this be so
As life is born from pain of birth
As night begets the dawn
Joy will follow pain.

—Darrell Stoddard

⊢⊣

"*Ye cannot behold with your natural eyes, for the present time, the design of your God concerning those things which shall come hereafter, and the glory which shall follow after much tribulation. For after much tribulation come the blessings.*"

(*Doctrine and Covenants*, p. 104)

Appendixes

—

The Author

Darrell Stoddard, a board certified auricular therapist, is a champion for long-lasting alternatives to Western pain treatments. He has researched pain for the past fifteen years and administered over eighteen thousand treatments of auricular and bioelectrical therapy, mostly at the Freedom Center for Advanced Medicine in Provo, Utah. In 1997, he founded the Pain Research Institute, a worldwide network of doctors that contribute to and maintain a website dedicated to non-surgical and non-drug pain prevention and relief.

—•—

The Pain Research Institute

The Pain Research Institute, founded in 1997, is a worldwide network of doctors who are dedicated to, philosophically supportive of, and contribute to the pain research conducted by the founder, Darrell Stoddard, a board certified auricular therapist. The primary function of the organization is to communicate urgent advances in research on pain treatment without surgery or drugs. The Institute website is filled with articles, tips on pain prevention, and the latest information on treating pain without surgery or drugs. More information can be found at *www.healpain.net.*

—

Directions for Applying
Biotape™

Dehydration is the number one cause of non-injury and non-impact injury pain. As many as seventy to eighty percent of all adults are dehydrated. It is vital for almost anyone in pain to drink more water along with using the tape. Electricity will not travel through dry tissue! (Distilled water will not conduct an electrical signal, and reverse osmosis water is a poor conductor.) Most exercise and non-impact work injuries occur when people are dehydrated. Such injuries could be cut in less than half if people would drink more water.

Biotape™ may not work on those who are dehydrated or who are taking diuretics. Also, if you are drinking city water, you should let your water sit out, uncovered, for a minimum of two hours, but preferably overnight to allow the chlorine to evaporate. Chlorine is a necessary germicide in our water, but it is also a toxin. Chlorine kills houseplants and goldfish, it killed my bonsai trees, and the Nazis used it in their gas chambers to exterminate human beings. The good news is that it costs nothing to get rid of the chlorine. It takes only a little planning.

Before applying Biotape™, always shave or clip your hair, if you have any where the tape will be applied. Clean the area with rubbing alcohol to remove dry skin and skin oils. This will help the tape to stick better. Then remove the white liner from the tape. The diagrams that follow show suggested placements found to be most effective.

General Rule

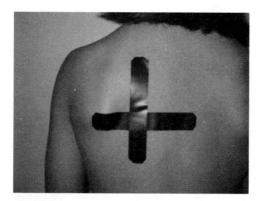

A general rule to follow when applying Biotape™ is to run a $4^1/_2$-inch strip through the pain area and another $4^1/_2$-inch strip crossing at right angles over any trigger points (points that are especially tender when palpitated). There is no right or wrong way to apply the tape other than to place the tape over the pain area.

Headache Pain

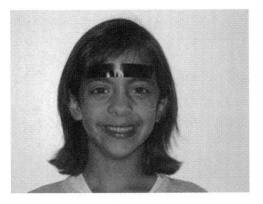

Apply a strip from temple to temple across the forehead just above the eyebrows. If necessary, apply another strip around the back of the neck as close to the skull as possible. (Hair may need to be removed.)

Low Back Pain

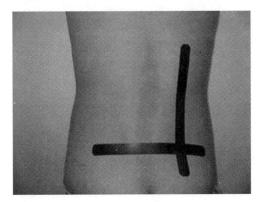

Apply a single vertical strip along side the lumbar spine, on the side that hurts most, over the sacroiliac (S.I.) joint (where the dimple is). The patient should bend forward a little as the tape is applied. Another horizontal strip should then be applied across both S.I. joints. If the S.I. joint is not the most tender spot on the low back (eight-five percent of the time it *is* this joint), run the horizontal strip across the most tender point instead of, or in addition to, running it over the S.I. joints.

Shoulder Pain

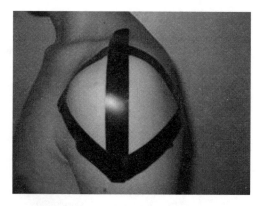

Apply a single, 9-inch strip over the top of the shoulder and about 4 inches down the arm. Add another strip at right angles to the first, over the shoulder joint. If the pain is at the point of the shoulder, a third strip is applied around the point of the shoulder.

Knee Pain

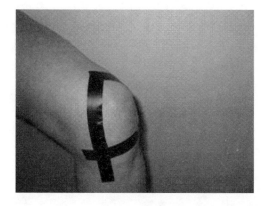

For knee pain, taping around the kneecap and joint (not around the leg) while the knee is bent at a 90-degree angle seems to work best. Use one strip about 9 inches long on each side of the knee joint, with the strips connecting above the kneecap. Place a third strip horizontally below the kneecap, connecting the other two strips. When finished it will look like the capital letter "A."

Foot Pain

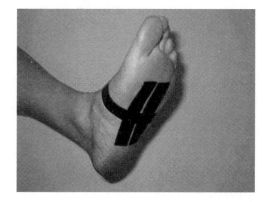

For peripheral neuropathy and pain or burning on the bottom of the foot, place two or three strips side by side along the bottom of the foot. While the patient puts weight on the foot, place another strip around the foot, joining it over the instep. If weight is not on the foot, the tape will be too tight when the patient stands.

Elbow Pain

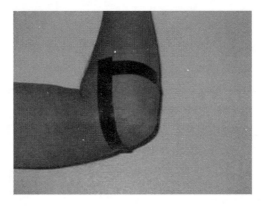

For elbow pain, the tape should be applied on the outside of the elbow with the elbow bent. If applied while the arm is straight, the tape will pull off when the arm is bent.

Finger Pain

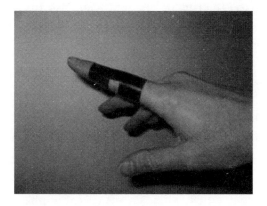

For arthritic fingers or finger pain, place the tape along and around the fingers.

Carpal Tunnel or Wrist Pain

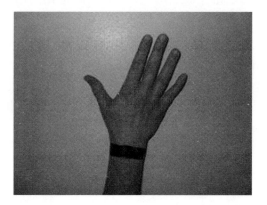

Place a single strip around the wrist at the joint.

Scars

It is also effective to place tape across any scars that may be blocking electrical signals.

Acupuncture

For those familiar with acupuncture, the tape can be placed along acupuncture meridians. One strip of Biotape™ toward the end of the meridian increases the signal (Chi) going through the entire meridian more effectively than acupuncture needles. This is a measurable phenomenon.

Other Considerations

Biotape™ may not work for someone on pain medication. Pain medication suppresses signals to the brain. Biotape™ is applied to reconnect the broken circuits that cause pain. One modality may work against the other.

As with any kind of tape, some people may find themselves allergic to the adhesive on the Biotape™, or to the Biotape™ itself. Some itching under the tape is normal; it should be expected. However, if the user develops a rash or blisters, the tape should be removed. Even if it has only been possible to use the tape for one day, some healing is to be expected. If no allergic reaction results, the tape should be left on for as long as possible, or until the desired results are achieved.

If the tape begins to come off, you can tack it down with any other type of tape intended for use on the skin. Paper surgical tape is a good choice and stays on surprisingly well in water. Biotape ™ will continue to conduct signals as long as it touches the skin—even if the adhesive is no longer viable. Thus Biotape™ can be used over and over again.

Biotape™ can be left on while showering or bathing. Simply be careful not to scrub it off. Pat your skin dry instead of rubbing it. Placing waterproof tape over the Biotape™ while showering or bathing will also help it adhere even in water.

The body knows how to heal itself. When the body does not heal, either the messages from the broken circuits are not getting to the brain or the signal is not returning to the cells to tell them how to repair and replicate. Biotape™, we believe, can help the body accomplish both functions if it is left on long enough.

No medical claims are made for Biotape™. The manufacturer has made it available solely for research purposes. The information given above is only theoretical until established by double-blind, placebo-controlled studies. This information should be applied to human beings with the intention of making a diagnosis, treating or preventing disease, or restoring, correcting, or modifying physiological function.

Because we are a research organization, we would like to learn about your success or failure using Biotape™ to relieve pain. We need your input. Please write (e-mail) to stoddard@healpain.net and tell us about your experience with Biotape™.

Darrell J. Stoddard, Founder
Pain Research Institute
http://www.healpain.net

—•—

Where to Obtain Biotape™ and Biotape™ Hydration Formula

There is currently only one source where these products are available for consumer use.

Smart Inventions, Inc.

6319 E. Alondra Blvd.,

Paramount,

CA 90723-3750

Ph Toll Free 1-800-977-6336